LIVING WIT' RHEUN

PHILIPPA PIGACHE has been a journalist and writer
for more than thirty years, starting on local newspapers
and women's magazines, moving to national newspapers, radio and television and, more recently, becoming
a freelance medical science writer. She has worked on
the *Sunday Times*, *Daily Mail* and *Guardian*, and for ITN
and BBC science features.

She started to specialize in writing about medicine
chiefly because she was married to a doctor. (Her own
educational background is in modern languages and the
theatre.) She has contributed to consumer health pages
and journals for health professionals for twenty years and
has won awards for her medical journalism and also for
her fiction. She is currently the honorary secretary of the
Medical Journalists' Association and editor of their
journal, the *MJA News*.

She has written consumer health books on arthritis and
Attention Deficit Hyperactivity Disorder (ADHD). She
has two children, three grandchildren and three cats. She
lives in Sussex and paints and gardens in her spare time.

Overcoming Common Problems Series

Selected titles
A full list of titles is available from Sheldon Press,
36 Causton Street, London SW1P 4ST, and on our website at
www.sheldonpress.co.uk

Assertiveness: Step by Step
Dr Windy Dryden and Daniel Constantinou

Body Language at Work
Mary Hartley

The Cancer Guide for Men
Helen Beare and Neil Priddy

The Candida Diet Book
Karen Brody

The Chronic Fatigue Healing Diet
Christine Craggs-Hinton

Cider Vinegar
Margaret Hills

Comfort for Depression
Janet Horwood

Confidence Works
Gladeana McMahon

Coping Successfully with Hay Fever
Dr Robert Youngson

Coping Successfully with Pain
Neville Shone

Coping Successfully with Panic Attacks
Shirley Trickett

Coping Successfully with Prostate Cancer
Dr Tom Smith

Coping Successfully with Prostate Problems
Rosy Reynolds

Coping Successfully with RSI
Maggie Black and Penny Gray

Coping Successfully with Your Hiatus Hernia
Dr Tom Smith

Coping with Alopecia
Dr Nigel Hunt and Dr Sue McHale

Coping with Anxiety and Depression
Shirley Trickett

Coping with Blushing
Dr Robert Edelmann

Coping with Bronchitis and Emphysema
Dr Tom Smith

Coping with Candida
Shirley Trickett

Coping with Childhood Asthma
Jill Eckersley

Coping with Chronic Fatigue
Trudie Chalder

Coping with Coeliac Disease
Karen Brody

Coping with Cystitis
Caroline Clayton

Coping with Depression and Elation
Dr Patrick McKeon

Coping with Down's Syndrome
Fiona Marshall

Coping with Dyspraxia
Jill Eckersley

Coping with Eczema
Dr Robert Youngson

Coping with Endometriosis
Jo Mears

Coping with Epilepsy
Fiona Marshall and
Dr Pamela Crawford

Coping with Fibroids
Mary-Claire Mason

Coping with Gallstones
Dr Joan Gomez

Coping with Gout
Christine Craggs-Hinton

Coping with a Hernia
Dr David Delvin

Coping with Incontinence
Dr Joan Gomez

Coping with Long-Term Illness
Barbara Baker

Coping with the Menopause
Janet Horwood

Coping with a Mid-life Crisis
Derek Milne

Coping with Polycystic Ovary Syndrome
Christine Craggs-Hinton

Coping with Psoriasis
Professor Ronald Marks

Overcoming Common Problems Series

Overcoming Common Problems Series

Overcoming Common Problems

Living with Rheumatoid Arthritis

Philippa Pigache

sheldon**PRESS**

First published in Great Britain in 2005

Sheldon Press
36 Causton Street
London SW1P 4ST

The author and publisher have made every effort to ensure that the external website
and email addresses included in this book are correct and up to date at the time of
going to press. The author and publisher are not responsible for the content, quality
or continuing accessibility of the sites.

British Library Cataloguing-in-Publication Data

A catalogue record for this book is available from the British Library

ISBN 0–85969–933–1

1 3 5 7 9 10 8 6 4 2

Typeset by Deltatype Limited, Birkenhead, Merseyside
Printed in Great Britain by Ashford Colour Printers

To Elizabeth,
who is brave and beautiful and funny
despite enduring more than twenty years with RA

Contents

Introduction

All illness starts with some symptom or other, and, usually, rheumatoid arthritis starts as pain. Only when you get to a doctor do those symptoms acquire a name: a diagnosis. When you have a pain the first thing you ask yourself is, 'Is it normal? Is it one of the usual aches and pains that come and go during life, or is it something serious? Something I should take to the doctor?'

The names used for the aches and pains that flesh is heir to vary throughout history, and are also affected by fashion. 'Rheumatism' is so generally applied to pain, stiffness and discomfort as to be almost meaningless. Fifty years ago almost any old person would say they suffered from rheumatics, or possibly lumbago (from the lumbar region of the spine, which is the most common site for backache). More recently 'neuralgia' (nerve pain) or 'sciatica' (from a particular nerve in the hip) became fashionable, and still later almost everyone's backache was attributed to a 'slipped disc'. These days 'arthritis' is the word widely used to describe pain and stiffness in joints – it actually means inflammation of the joints, and let's face it, inflammation is usually painful – unless, that is, you are a sportsman, and then you probably say you suffer from 'cartilage problems'.

The fact is that it is perfectly normal to suffer from pain and stiffness of the joints from time to time, especially as the body gets older. Physical change can take place without someone becoming ill, disabled or even noticeably aware of it. The most common form of arthritis, the kind called *osteo*arthritis (*osteo* meaning bone, one of the several materials joints are made of), is almost inevitable if you live long enough.

But the disease called rheumatoid arthritis (RA hereon for short) is not normal, has nothing to do with ageing – children also suffer – and it is not something anyone should be expected to cope with alone, without everything modern medicine and therapy can offer by way of help.

To be diagnosed with RA can be a terrible shock. You don't just have the pain and stiffness, you feel generally ill (malaise) and, above all, you learn you have something that is never completely cured: a *chronic* illness – one that may come and go and possibly be with you for the rest of your life (though, of course, it may not). You learn that it could permanently damage your joints and make it difficult, if not impossible, to do things you have taken for granted – sleeping, even. It is unsurprising that being diagnosed with RA can make people wretched, not to say downright depressed.

People react in different ways to being told that they have a chronic illness. They may go into denial, try to carry on as normal, ignoring the symptoms even when they are acute, resisting treatment and pretending nothing has changed or needs to be done. They may put blind faith in their doctor and leave all decisions to him, preferring to be spared all explanation and especially grisly detail of what is happening in their body. On the other hand, on discovering that total cure is not on the agenda with prescribed medicines, they may rush from alternative practitioner, to health-store, to internet site trying out questionable cures which claim to have worked miraculously in some cases (though probably not published with chapter and verse) in a desperate search for just anything that may help. Others become their illness: it becomes not an unpleasant addition to their lives, but their entire existence, their only interest and topic of conversation.

But some people react to the knowledge by deciding to take charge. They want to know all there is to know about it, to become experts in the nature and management of their condition and partners with those who can help them. Not so that it dominates them, but so that they may dominate the illness. Studies show that people who have some understanding of their illness cope better with a chronic condition.

Knowledge puts you in charge. By understanding the disease you begin to take control of it. You develop realistic expectations which help you overcome fear and anxiety. The unknown creates anxiety and uncertainty, stress. This is partly because in the absence of information the imagination creates disaster scenarios more lurid than reality. The truth then becomes reassuring.

What's more, informed patients communicate better with the health professionals they deal with; they share decisions on their treatment. And since no one knows your body as well as you do, by using knowledge to monitor your condition and progress you make a unique contribution to tailoring your therapeutic programme to your particular needs. And RA is slightly different for each person –

recognizably the same animal, but with variations in colouring, features and emphasis.

Take courage. Much can be done to relieve the symptoms and prevent the worst ravages of RA. With the help of the right drugs, doctors, therapists and a therapeutic life-style, not to mention a supportive family and friends, you can beat this, or at the very least keep the beast in its place. This book is designed to help you rise above RA.

Hints for the reader

If you wish, you can read this book from beginning to end. Or you could take a skip and a jump, or simply dip in and out, picking out what interests or concerns you. Only the first three chapters, which explain the basic anatomy of joints and what rheumatoid arthritis is all about, are important for understanding much of what comes after. There are cross-headings and titles to help you find your way around the text. Difficult words are explained in the text and those printed in *italic type* when first they appear (though not throughout the text) are also listed in the glossary at the end of the book. Information that is not essential to understanding the general story of rheumatoid arthritis is sometimes picked out in special boxes.

Part 1: About RA

1

Rheumatoid arthritis: the who, where, why and what

Let's start with the name: the word 'arthritis' comes from the Greek words for a joint – *arthron* (also found in *arti*culate – join-up) – and inflammation – *itis*. Just to confuse you, arthritis does not invariably involve inflammation, although the rheumatoid variety does. For this reason some doctors prefer the term *arthropathy*, which is more precise, meaning joint disease. The term 'arthritis' covers many different conditions that affect the joints and different parts of joints.

The 'rheumatoid' part of the name has a long and varied history. The Greek word *rheum* means flow, and describes diseases which pass through many organs of the body (what doctors call *systemic*). This is what the French phrase *être enrhumé* for having a cold implies, and when Shakespeare speaks of 'a rheum in mine eye' he is being even more literal and means that tears are flowing. More recently, English people have come to use the words 'rheumatism' or 'rheumatics' to stand for the aches and pains that accompany a cold, or ageing.

However, when 'rheumatoid' and 'arthritis' appear together they have a very specific meaning. They are the name of a condition that affects particular joints – freely movable, multi-directional ones – although, since the illness is systemic (it affects the whole body) it affects other organs too. Some of the symptoms of rheumatoid arthritis (and we will simplify life by referring to it as RA) are the same as those that occur in other forms of arthritis and some are quite distinct.

There are a number of theories as to what causes the disease, but most experts believe it originates with *antibodies*, part of the body's defence system, produced to attack foreign invaders like bacteria or viruses, making a mistake and attacking the body's own tissues: what is known as an *auto-immune disease*. (You can look up these and other medical terms in the glossary at the end of the book.)

1

The multiple personality of arthritis

To know what RA is, it is useful to know what it is not. There are more than 100 types of arthritis, some of them blessedly rare. As we have explained, not all forms of arthritis involve inflammation or inflammation alone. Nevertheless, everyone with arthritis experiences three common sets of symptoms:

- warmth, pain, soreness, tenderness or irritation (variously described forms of discomfort) accompanied by swelling and redness in one or more joints;
- stiffness in the joint, especially on waking or after inactivity;
- difficulty or pain in moving the joint which results in loss of movement and flexibility.

But although these many forms of arthritis cause common problems, they arise from different processes and affect different joints. It is possible to group them under their principal cause.

Wear and tear or degenerative arthritis

This group includes the most common form of arthritis, *osteoarthritis* (OA) – *osteon* is Greek for bone – or degenerative joint disease (DJD), which has the advantage of being plain English but the disadvantage of suggesting that only the elderly suffer from it. It is worth knowing about OA because it is so widespread – 90 per cent of people will develop it to some degree if they live long enough – that many RA sufferers may also develop OA just to complicate the picture.

Joints, like the moving parts of a motor car or washing machine, perform less reliably with heavy use or the passage of time. The exact moment that they start to give trouble will depend partly on the quality of the basic components but also on the stresses and strains to which they have been subjected and the care with which they have been maintained.

In human terms this means that when you develop OA, or less probably *whether* you develop it, depends on several things. You may have been born with joints containing the kind of *cartilage* that gets thin and flaky with age, or suffer the not uncommon misfortune of being born with two legs not of exactly the same length. There again, you may have hammered your joints in sport or athletics (footballer's knee, or athlete's back) or because you have exposed them to the excessive strain of carrying around too much body weight. All these things contribute to OA because the cartilage that lines the bones of our joints can be damaged and also degenerates with time and use, the bones thicken and the joints become stiff. Inflammation may also occur, although it is not the cause of the condition. OA occurs in a large number of joints, not only freely moving ones but also in the spine, and is most common in the load-bearing joints that take the strain of carrying our bodies around.

A break-down in body chemistry

Everyone has heard of *gout*, and most of us know it affects chiefly the big toe and occasionally other joints in the feet. Inflammation plays a role in this sort of arthritis: inflammation caused by the body producing too much of a chemical called *uric acid* from which crystals form inside the tissues of the joint causing the inflammation, swelling and excruciating pain. There is a similar, less severe kind of gout known as *pseudo* (false*) gout* in which the body makes calcium phosphate crystals in the cartilage lining the joints.

Inflammation

As we have seen, inflammation plays a part in many forms of arthritis. In RA a malfunction of the inflammatory process is at the root of the condition. RA affects fewer joints than OA: the freely moving joints of the hand, feet, knees, hips and neck. It is the most common of the inflammatory arthrites, affecting between 2 and 3 per cent of the population worldwide.

Another form of inflammatory arthritis is the dauntingly named *ankylosing spondylitis* of the spine (from Greek words for stiffening, for vertebrae – the joints of the spine – and for inflammation). Included in the inflammation group are a number of kinds of arthritis that involve a reaction to infection: *Reiter's disease* in which the eyes become inflamed; *psoriatic arthritis* (part of the skin condition psoriasis made famous in the Dennis Potter television serial *The Singing Detective)*; *systemic lupus erythematosus* (another skin and joint disease); *colitic arthritis* (in which the *colon*, part of the digestive tract, is affected) and last, but not least, *Lyme disease* (not Greek this time, but named after a place in Connecticut, USA, where it was first described). This is passed on via a tick bite and has sometimes been confused with RA because it produces similar symptoms, including those affecting the joints. Fortunately it occurs only in areas where the particular carrier-tick lives.

Box 1 on pp. 6–7 gives a brief history of RA.

N.B. No form of arthritis is infectious or contagious, and having one kind does not predispose you to developing another.

Who develops rheumatoid arthritis?

The common view is that the incidence of RA in the population is constantly the same the world over at between 2 and 3 per cent of the population. This rate has recently shown signs of a decline, and slight variations in certain populations have been detected. As many as 5.3 per cent of Native Americans may have RA, and it appears to be slightly less common among black South Africans, the Chinese and among Japanese women (as low as 0.1 per cent).

We are usually told that RA is just as common in cities as it is in the countryside. But there is some evidence from recent studies of the Chinese that not only is it generally less common in that country, but that villagers are even less likely to develop it than city dwellers. This cannot be entirely explained by the fact that rural populations generally have poorer access to doctors and are therefore less likely to report illness.

The major discrepancy in the incidence of RA is, however, between the sexes. For every one man, three women develop the disease. Not only are women more likely to get it, they generally get it sooner and they get it worse. RA does occur in children, but more typically it shows up first for women in their thirties and for men in their forties. Incidence increases in both sexes to a peak in the mid-fifties. The longer someone has the disease, the worse the symptoms are likely to become.

Caitlin's story
Caitlin lives with her parents in Canberra, Australia. When she was only a few months old her parents became worried because they noticed that her knees were red and swollen. Caitlin was taken into hospital for a few days with what the doctors first thought was 'a virus', but several months later, when the results

4

of all the tests had come back, they gave her shattered parents the diagnosis: Caitlin had juvenile RA.

Caitlin is now nine years old. She still has the RA in her knees, toes and wrist joints. But she doesn't let it get in her way at school. She does everything her classmates do, loves playing football and goes skiing with her family every season. She has to take anti-inflammatory medication to help make her joints less stiff, particularly in the mornings, and because this alone was insufficient to control the inflammation she was referred to a specialist rheumatologist who prescribed methotrexate, a drug used to treat moderate to severe RA, which she takes once a week. It makes Caitlin rather sick so she also takes folic acid to help alleviate the nausea and vomiting.

'I have folic acid every night,' says Caitlin, 'and on Saturday nights I take the methotrexate. I used to take it on Thursday, but then I was too sick to go to my football training, so I'm taking it on Saturdays now.' Caitlin also goes to hydrotherapy classes at the Canberra Hospital every Tuesday, where she does exercises to help her joints.

Why does someone develop RA?

There is no simple answer to what causes RA. It's not part of normal ageing, like osteoarthritis. It's not a result of something we eat or pick up from the environment. It's not passed from one person to another by some infectious organism, nor is it passed down from parents to children in the genes like *haemophilia* (when someone's blood lacks the factor that makes it clot) – although more of genes later.

About the most we can say is that at least we understand more about RA than they did 150 years ago, when doctors used to bleed patients for this and a wide range of conditions because they had so few proven effective treatments available. We now know that in RA part of the inflammatory process, which normally clocks in to protect the body from damage or infection, for some reason runs amok and turns against the healthy tissues of the joints and, if unchecked, destroys them. But what makes one person's system do this and not another's?

Box 1   *A brief history of rheumatoid arthritis*

Some people have blamed RA on modern life: living in crowded cities, eating junk food and being exposed to high levels of pollution. But there is clear evidence that this is not so. Joints of mammals damaged by arthritis have been found dating from prehistoric times.

4500 BC

The earliest physical evidence of RA found in skeletons of Native Americans discovered in Tennessee, USA.

400 BC

The father of medicine, the Greek philosopher–physician Hippocrates writes the first description of RA. He uses the word 'rheums', not in Shakespeare's sense of wet, or runny, but to indicate the disease flowing between joints.

123 BC

An Indian text called *Caraka Samhita* describes a disease where swollen, painful joints strike first the hands and feet, then spread to the body, causing loss of appetite, and occasionally fever.

AD 1591

The first book describing RA: a French physician called Guillaume de Baillou uses the term *rheumatism* for a condition characterized by inflammation, soreness, stiffness in the muscles, and pain in and around the joints. 'The whole body hurts, in some the face is flushed; pain is most severe around the joints ... At night ... the pain becomes more serious and the patient cannot sleep.'

1680

Thomas Sydenham, an English physician, treats 'rheumatism' with a Peruvian bark now known to contain the anti-malarial agent quinine. (Today a modern anti-malarial, hydroxychloroquine sulfate, is used to treat RA.)

1763

Willow bark is first used as treatment. It contains *salicylate*, the pain-killing, anti-inflammatory ingredient in aspirin still used to treat all forms of arthritis. At this time there is little understanding of the causes of the disease and it is frequently treated, like many other conditions, by bleeding the patient.

1859

Sir Alfred Garrod, a London physician, coins the clinical term *rheumatoid arthritis*; the first reference appears in medical literature.

1893

The first joint replacement surgery is performed by a surgeon called W. A. Lane using a system of carbon-steel screws and plates.

1897

The Bayer Company isolates the active ingredient in willow bark and starts manufacturing acetylsalicylic acid, better known as aspirin. It rapidly becomes the standard treatment for pain and rheumatic disorders.

1912

US physician Frank Billings suggests that RA and other systemic diseases may be a response to localized infection.

1929

Another pain-killing drug still in use emerges: the periodic injection of gold salts.

1939

Australian researcher Sir McFarlane Burnet proposes that RA could be an auto-immune disease: one in which the body's defence system malfunctions and attacks its own healthy tissues. The theory is still held to be true today.

1948

Two American doctors, Philip Hench and Edward Kendall, at the Mayo Clinic in Maryland, USA, establish the therapeutic anti-inflammatory effects of steroid hormones. The discovery will win them a Nobel Prize. Another milestone: an antibody called *rheumatoid factor* (RF) is identified in the blood of most people with RA.

There is almost certainly more than one cause: something that makes some people uniquely vulnerable in the first place, plus another factor, possibly more than one, that 'triggers' the illness in susceptible people. This composite picture of disease causation crops up more and more in modern medicine.

The genetic factor

Two types of evidence support the idea that people may inherit genes that make them more susceptible to RA. One is studies of twins: with identical twins – those whose genetic material (DNA) is identical – if one develops RA the other is nearly four times as likely to develop it than with non-identical twins, who share only as much DNA as siblings. But brothers and sisters of someone with RA have a higher than normal chance of developing the disease too, confirming the genetic component. Genes for susceptibility are often inherited, but on their own they don't cause the illness.

The other thing that supports the idea of some genetic vulnerability is the fact that people who share one variation in a particular part of the body's defence system – their *histocompatibility* group – appear to be more susceptible to RA than others. The immune system is designed to recognize and attack only foreign invaders like germs or tumours, but in RA, as we have seen, it goes wrong and starts attacking healthy joints. It's worth noting that certain histocompatibility *antigens* are more common in one ethnic group than another. This may go some way to explaining why Native Americans should be more susceptible and some Africans and Asians less so, bucking the predominant trend for incidence of the disease being otherwise consistent in populations worldwide.

A major study of families with RA is currently going on in America and Europe, organized by the North American Rheumatoid Arthritis Consortium, with the goal of finding which genes are shared by siblings who develop the disease but not by those who don't. These distinguishing genes, or pieces of genes, are known as *genetic markers*. If they could be identified it might be possible to know who is most at risk and so do something about preventing them developing the disease.

Environmental triggers and the infection connection

But what is different about the identical twins who *don't* both develop RA? The prevailing idea is that something in the environment triggers the disease, so that if both twins are genetically susceptible one cannot have been exposed to the trigger. And the most popular candidate as the trigger is thought to be some infection early in life. This theory is proposed as a possible cause for a number of diseases where the auto-immune system starts attacking the body's own tissues. The suggestion is that, faced with an infection, the immune system very properly gets to work to fight it but for some reason, when the infection is vanquished, instead of withdrawing, the immune system turns its guns on to healthy tissue. It is possible that in insulin-dependent diabetes, in leukaemia and in RA some quite unremarkable childhood infection flicks the switch and starts the antibodies off in the wrong direction.

Professor Alan Silman of the epidemiology unit at Manchester University points out that rates have declined since RA was first described some 200 years ago. Could this be explained by the fact that nowadays people are vaccinated and immunized against a number of childhood diseases? Could one of these infections – measles, mumps, rubella – more common in the past, have been the trigger to RA in susceptible people? Professor Silman quotes other hints of an infectious cause: a person who developed RA the day after having a yellow fever vaccine, a possible connection with one of the antigens in tetanus immunization, or the fact that cat-owners are more likely to develop the disease!

Mention of cats brings us to our familiar enemies, environmental pollutants. Eighty per cent of people with RA (and some who don't develop it) produce the characteristic antibody *rheumatoid factor* (RF). Usually the presence of RF in the blood predicts that the condition will be severe. A recent study discovered that those exposed to atmospheric pollutants like carbon dioxide (produced when we burn things), silica (fine industrial fibres), asbestos, and cigarette smoke have increased levels of RF in their blood. This supports the suggestion in the population statistics that those living in cities could be slightly more likely to develop RA.

Whatever the multiple causes turn out to be, the sleuths in medical research believe they have the scent of the RA fox in their nostrils. For a normally cautious profession, many researchers sound optimistic that the causes behind the rogue behaviour of antibodies in auto-immune diseases will be discovered in the near future and that then a cure, not just treatment, will become a real possibility.

2

What goes wrong in rheumatoid arthritis?

Understanding what goes wrong in a disease is easier if you know how the system works when it's all going right. The joints of the human skeleton are complex pieces of engineering. In an engine the moving parts are cushioned from shocks and wear and tear by bearings, lubricating fluids, springs and shock-absorbers. The joints of vertebrates (animals with a skeleton) have to withstand the friction of one part rubbing against another, the stress of bearing loads and the strain of muscles and ligaments pulling and contracting against them to achieve movement and maintain posture. They have the equivalent of bearings and lubricants though it is a great deal more complicated in a living system that grows, ages and repairs itself.

The human body has more than 100 joints. In the adult body many of these move little if at all and we are happily unaware of them. Joints are of three types. Some are rigid, like junctions between bone in the skull and in the pelvis. They are movable only in children, to allow for growth, and in special circumstances like pregnancy to accommodate delivering a baby. Joints like these are unaffected by RA.

Some joints are slightly mobile, like those between the vertebrae (segments or joints of the spine). In the spine each vertebra is separated from its neighbour by a little pad of cartilage called a disc. If these joints move more than a little and the disc becomes damaged or displaced a 'slipped disc' results. Certain kinds of arthritis – osteoarthritis or ankylosing spondylitis – may develop in the spine but it is not affected in RA.

The third kind of joint is a freely movable one. Ask someone to name a joint and they immediately think of this kind: hips, knee, wrist, ankle, shoulder or those in the hands and feet. These joints may be affected by RA. They are known as *synovial* (a Latin name coined by the medieval physician–philosopher Paracelsus) joints. Figures 1 (opposite) and 2 (p.12) show the different kinds of joints affected by OA and RA.

The anatomy of a synovial joint
We are inclined to take our bodies for granted until they go wrong. The complexity, beauty even, of the way joints have evolved to

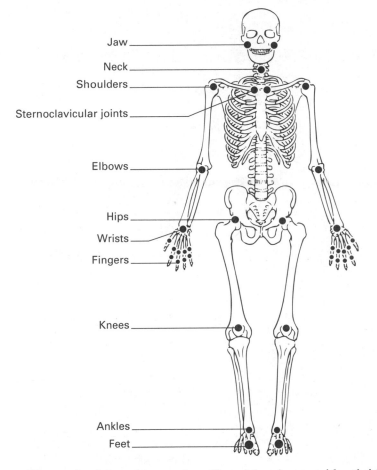

Figure 1   Joints that can be affected by rheumatoid arthritis

enable human beings to stand upright, twist, turn, bound, lift and do
subtle, co-ordinated actions like limbo-dancing or playing the piano
is actually quite breathtaking when you consider it in engineering
terms. The components of freely movable joints have complementary functions all of which play a part in the body's versatile
capacity for movement.

In a joint two or more bones meet. **Bone** is a strong, durable
material. It supports the body's framework, but it is rigid and can
fracture under mechanical stress. Bone is a living material and in

11

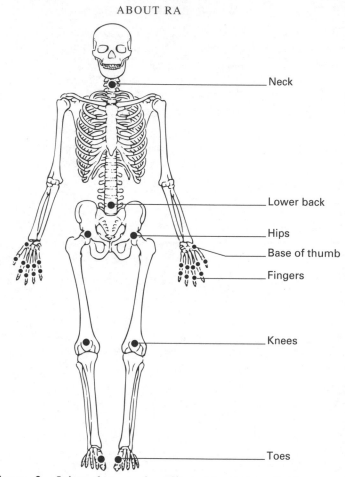

Figure 2   Joints that can be affected by osteoarthritis

youth it grows. Even when an adult has reached full height the living cells of bone continue to reproduce and replace themselves (see Box 2 on p.14 for more on bone cells). This process of cell replication, which in the healthy joint is completely balanced, becomes disrupted in RA.

Lining the bones of the joint, in a manner similar to soft metal bearings in an engine, is a cushion of material called **cartilage**. The smooth, slippery surface and compressibility of cartilage minimizes friction between the bones of the joint, and its spongy consistency enables it to take up fluid and nutrients produced inside the joint capsule. A sturdy framework of connective tissue fibres called *collagen* holds the cartilage together and gives it durability. The cartilage itself has no blood supply, which may limit its ability to heal when damaged.

Surrounding the bone endings lined with their protective cartilage coating is a tough, **fibrous capsule** full of fluid. It is a distinctive feature of freely movable joints that they are hermetically enclosed in this capsule. The moist lining of the capsule is called the **synovial membrane** and it produces clear, viscous **synovial fluid** that fills the joint, bathing all the moving parts rather like lubricating oil in an engine. RA starts in the synovial membrane and goes on to damage other parts of the joint.

There are other components of a synovial joint. **Ligaments** are cord-like structures that attach one bone to another across a joint, rather like guy ropes. They stabilize the joint and prevent it bending too far or in the wrong direction. For example, ligaments each side of the knee prevent it from moving to either side when bent or bending back on itself when fully extended.

Muscles have a number of roles. They generate the power required for movement, but they are also essential to stability, maintaining a joint in a steady position. For example, if you raise your arms above your head to comb your hair one group of muscles organizes the movement of your hands and wrists in combing while another holds your arms in their raised position. Muscles also provide protection to the joint; they play the role of shock-absorber. To realize this you only have to miss a step when running downstairs. Your muscles are unprepared for the sudden jolt and you feel the shock through your ankle and knee all the way to your hip. When a step, or more particularly a leap, is anticipated the appropriate muscles prepare to take the strain.

Muscles are attached to bone by **tendons**. They are to some extent similar to ligaments except that they connect muscle to bone rather than bone to bone. Tendons are extensions of muscles and move in conjunction with them when they tighten or contract. You can feel tendons tightening inside your elbow if you bend your arm, and they stand out like powerful hawsers at the back of the knee where they tether the ham-string muscles essential to standing upright and walking. Tendons are surrounded by an envelope called the **tendon sheath** which has a lining similar to the synovial membrane, making it easy to slide back and forth smoothly. This also can be affected in RA.

13

One other structure has a role in the joint. It is a little bag of fluid located between the muscle and the joint which acts like a cushion to facilitate the movement of muscle over the joint. It's called a **bursa**. This little sac can become inflamed if subjected to excessive or prolonged pressure. The condition is known to doctors as bursitis, but it also has a number of common-or-garden names derived from those who suffer from it: Housemaid's Knee, Tennis Elbow, and in the past, when weavers used to sit for hours on hard benches, Weaver's Bottom. Bursas are not affected by RA.

Box 2   *Osteoblasts and osteoclasts*

In some ways the body is like a river: it looks more or less the same over time, but the material it is composed of – in the case of a river, water; in the case of a human being, cells – is constantly changing. With a few exceptions the cells that make up the various organs of the body replace one another continuously in a kind of relay race throughout life: they mature, they grow old, they die, and new ones take their place. In bone, cell scavengers called osteoclasts break down and remove old bone. When they have done their job they either die or move on to another location. Meanwhile the bone that has become exposed attracts other bone cells called osteoblasts which lay down new bone.

Normally the amount of bone laid down matches perfectly the amount that is removed. But if there are too many osteoclasts or too few osteoblasts, then bone loss or osteoporosis occurs. In RA the main defect is that there are too many osteoclasts compared to normal bone.

What happens to joints in RA?

In describing what happens to the joints in someone with RA it is important to remember that there is wide variation in how people are affected. There is no standard programme for a chronic disease.

Some people suffer from a short bout of the illness affecting one or at most two joints and when it clears up appear to have sustained very little long-term damage. Others have repeated short bouts affecting different joints. Still others may have repeated or prolonged bouts of illness leaving their joints progressively worse every time, while for some people the disease starts and just goes on. The degree of permanent damage done to the joints is not apparent either to the patient or his doctors until it become severe.

The stages that a joint goes through as RA progresses are known from work with animals. But the stage the individual patient's joints have reached at the earlier stages of the illness is to some extent always going to be a calculated guess.

It all starts with inflammation

As we have explained, inflammation is designed to be a good thing. It is a sign that the body's immune system is at work repelling an invader – a germ – or healing damage. The symptoms of inflammation are the same wherever it goes on – a sore throat, a splinter, a corn or RA: warmth, redness, swelling and pain. The amount of inflammation, and hence the severity of the symptoms, is usually proportional to the severity of the injury or infection. It doesn't sound such a good thing put like that, but things that are good for you are often unpleasant while they do their work. Think of dieting and exercise. If you want more detail of the successful work of inflammation go to Box 3 opposite, 'Inflammation: the good news'.

Inflammation in RA

The inflammation of RA is a battle without an enemy; or possibly, to continue the metaphor, a battle that goes on after the enemy has been vanquished. The trigger for inflammation can be a virus, or something else that is foreign to the body – what is called an *antigen* because it generates 'anti' behaviour in the immune system. When the immune system recognizes a foreign invader it calls up increased numbers of two sorts of lymphocytes – T cells and B cells. Normally they target and destroy the antigens and inflammation then dies down. Not so in RA. For some reason the T and B cells become chronically 'overexcited'. One theory is that the communication between the cells of the immune system which is in the hands of those chemical messengers, the cytokines, is disturbed. The wrong message gets through and inflammation occurs with no apparent antigen – *Hamlet* without the ghost.

In RA the body launches a non-self-limiting immune response. In the absence of an antigen the body fights itself. This is why RA is classified as an auto-immune disease. Inflammation turned against the body itself is very far from a good thing.

15

Box 3 *Inflammation: the good news*

The body is a self-maintaining, self-repairing organism. Inflammation is an early sign of the defensive armoury of the immune system going into action to fight disease and repair damage.

There are a number of weapons in this armoury, each of which works in a slightly different way or against different forms of attack. White cells are the foot soldiers of the immune system. The ones active in inflammation are *lymphocytes* (the name indicates cells produced in the *lymph* glands, among other places), *neutrophils* (the meaning of this name relates to how the cells stain when prepared for going under a microscope) and *macrophages* (this one is rather fun: it's Greek for 'big eater' and describes how it goes about its work). They communicate with each other by chemical messengers called *cytokines* (meaning, literally, cell-mover).

Damaged cells at the site of infection or injury send an alarm call of chemical messengers that summons the foot soldiers. The blood supply to the battlefield is increased, producing redness and warmth. Clear fluid and white cells pass through the walls of the blood vessels into the surrounding tissues, causing swelling plus pain as a result of the pressure upon the surrounding tissues. While the fluid dilutes poisons and is mildly antiseptic, the white cells begin to engulf, break down and remove any foreign particles like bacteria that they encounter, cleaning up the battlefield so that reconstruction can begin. The fluid – called *inflammatory exudate* – has the same capacity as blood to clot and it will seal off clean wounds, like those resulting from a surgical operation, or minor infection. The clot sticks the edges of the wound together so that new tissue can grow to heal the breach.

If the enemy is not swiftly routed pus may form, composed of inflammatory exudate and broken-down cells of dead bacteria and white cells. (You may need to blow your nose, cough, or lance an abscess to clear this.) The bone-marrow and other blood-forming tissues are stimulated to produce more white cells; antibodies are formed tailored to target particular bacteria and harmful products. The body's temperature rises while the battle rages. In the normal course of events inflammation is ultimately self-limiting and disappears once the infection is cleared or the wound healed.

The progression of RA

Figure 3 overleaf shows the five stages of RA.

Stage 1

At this stage people have no symptoms and their joints appear completely normal. There is nothing but a susceptibility to the illness – indicated by an unknown genetic marker. A marker alone doesn't cause the disease but the vulnerability lies there, dormant.

Stage 2

This is the stage at which people experience the first symptoms of RA. Lymphocytes and macrophages produced by the immune system begin to congregate in the synovial lining of the joint capsule, sending out cytokines (chemical messengers) that cause it to become inflamed – *synovitis*. Increased numbers of two specific cytokines known to promote inflammation, *tumour necrosis factor* (TNF) and *interleukin-1* (IL-1) have been found in the joints of people with RA. (Other cytokines including other interleukins – there are more than 13 different ones – are produced that should damp down inflammation, but in RA these are outnumbered.) Cytokines also increase the number of blood vessels going to the synovium causing it to become warm, and cytokines leaking into the bloodstream may also explain the fatigue associated with this stage of RA. Other cytokines stimulate the production of various other substances that cause swelling, warmth and pain. These cytokines are a primary target for drugs that treat RA.

At Stage 2 the B lymphocytes undergo a transformation. They become another type of white blood cell called a plasma cell and start manufacturing antibodies in vast quantities. Antibodies are not normally present in the body. They are produced specifically to fight foreign invaders like bacteria or viruses. One particular antibody is so often found in the blood of people with RA that it is called *rheumatoid factor* (RF). The presence of RF in the blood is clear confirmation that someone has contracted RA. Confusingly, a few people have RA and no RF is detected.

Stage 3

At this stage the joint becomes so overcrowded with the extra cells from the immune system that its lining – the synovium – begins to change. It thickens up and its texture becomes spongy, a condition

17

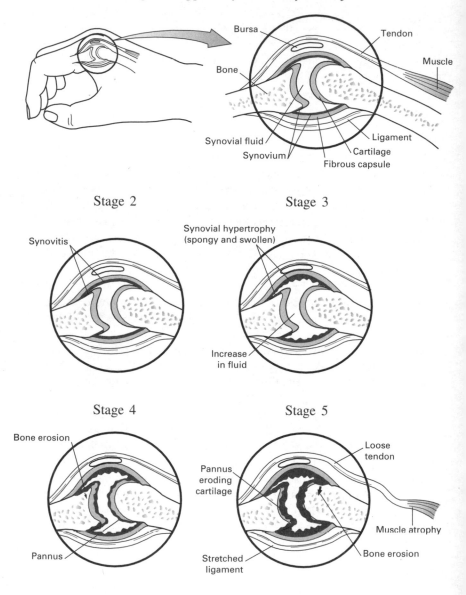

Figure 3 The stages of rheumatoid arthritis

known as *hypertrophy* (Greek for greater shape). The sheer volume of synovial fluid in the joint causes increasing stiffness and restriction of movement. The quantity of lubricating substance in the synovial fluid also increases, and its tendency to 'gel' is thought to cause the aggravated stiffness in the joint after a night in bed or a lengthy period sitting still.

Up to this stage someone with RA may feel pretty ill and will have had to endure all the uncomfortable symptoms of joint inflammation – pain, heat, swelling, stiffness and loss of movement. Nevertheless, no permanent damage has been done. Treatment may be able to halt and even reverse the course of the disease.

Stage 4

If RA progresses to this stage the inflamed synovium, initially the lining of the joint capsule, spreads up and over the cartilage that protects the ends of bone in the joint. This new growth is called a *pannus* (Latin for a coverlet). The pannus releases *enzymes* which begin to attack the cartilage. Other destructive enzymes are released by neutrophils (a variety of white blood cell) that have built up in the synovial fluid. Enzymes are organic substances that transform things, from a Greek word that means 'leavening', like yeast. Many enzymes play a constructive role in the body, but not in this particular case. Having destroyed or weakened the protective cartilage layer, they go on to eat away at the bone underneath the cartilage, creating tiny pits or *erosions*. The most vulnerable point is the edge of the cartilage around the neck of the bone ending.

Stage 5

If unchecked, enzymes produced by the pannus may damage the cartilage so badly that it ceases to cushion the bones of the joint and smooth movement becomes impossible. The patient may even feel the bones grating when the joint is moved. Doctors doing a physical examination can feel it too. At this stage, when the cartilage inside the capsule is totally eroded, the swelling of the joint may start to affect ligaments and tendons too, causing them to stretch so that they no longer hold the joint firm and it becomes wobbly. Muscles, weak through lack of use, begin to shrink (*atrophy*, Greek for losing their shape). Weakened and unstable, the joint no longer behaves predictably. And then, ironically, when the cartilage is effectively a write-off, the inflammation and the swelling often decrease, producing what is known as a 'burnt-out' joint. Now, as the swelling goes down, the stretched ligaments and tendons have become too loose to be much use in supporting the damaged joint.

The good news is that with modern intervention with drugs, only a small percentage of patients, perhaps less than 5 per cent, ever reach the disabling Stage 5 of RA.

Martin's story

Martin had developed insulin-dependent diabetes while still a young man. But he was otherwise healthy, active and in the prime of life and he rapidly took the irksome ritual of blood-sugar tests and insulin injections in his stride and carried on his life as normal. Sadly in his forties things began to go wrong in his life. He lost his job, began to drink too much and finally his marriage fell apart. Depressed and run down, his immune system let him down again (this kind of diabetes is an auto-immune disease). The joints of his fingers and wrists became so stiff and swollen he could not hold a pencil. His shoulders and ankles began to hurt too and he felt so tired he couldn't get out of bed. He lost his appetite, his insulin balance went haywire and he ended up in hospital where they diagnosed RA and began to treat it. For weeks, nearly months, Martin was really ill, but gradually the acute attack subsided and the joints of his hands returned to normal. He began to re-build his life. Ten years later Martin is thankfully able to cross his fingers that RA has not returned. The only permanent damage is to his right shoulder: his life as a spin-bowler is over.

3

The course of RA is a bumpy road with blind turnings

In the first chapters of this book we have considered RA from the outside: as observers. Even viewed objectively, with medical insight and hindsight it is a shifting and contradictory picture. It's an illness that may be over in weeks if you're lucky, or with you for the rest of your life if you're not. It may creep up on you stealthily or strike you down at one blow. It may spoil your tennis service or it may confine you to a wheel-chair. In the past, people accepted that illness was unexpected and unpredictable, handed down from on high. But today we expect doctors to tell us what will happen, how long it will last, what we can do about it. We want to know the future course of the illness, the *prognosis* (Greek again: to know in advance or predict) and hopefully, the cure.

If you have just been diagnosed with RA, or if you have lived with it coming and going for some time, as a twenty-first-century patient you naturally want answers to these questions. With a chronic and unpredictable illness like RA, that puts doctors (and authors) in a predicament. It is a good thing for a patient to have knowledge, including knowing of the possibility of a bad outcome. But it's good for patients to be optimistic: feeling doomed does not aid recovery or fight-back. To benefit from knowing what *might* happen people with RA must constantly remind themselves, 'It may not happen to me.'

What are the warning signs?

In Chapter 2 we described Stage 1 of RA: no symptoms, but a sleeping genetic susceptibility to developing RA that could be triggered at any moment. No one can say confidently how many lucky people carry that sleeping susceptibility to their graves without knowing about it. It is quite possible that we are all genetically susceptible to a number of illnesses but don't develop them because we are not exposed to an environmental trigger.

21

First symptoms

If and when RA is triggered, symptoms usually emerge gradually, starting with pain and stiffness in any of the joints shown on p. 11. Most people notice symptoms first in the hands, or maybe the ankles or toes. Swelling may not be obvious to begin with, but as the pain increases and persists swelling appears in the joints, usually within a month of the first symptoms being noted. Very exceptionally swelling follows pain a year or more later.

But some have a different experience. They may become aware of general stiffness, particularly first thing in the morning; or they may notice increasingly pronounced joint swelling but with no pain to begin with. Others suffer bouts of swelling and/or pain which flares up and then disappears almost as quickly. A few older patients experience first symptoms as stiff and aching muscles in the hips or shoulders. Finally, there is the bowl-you-over, rapid onset manifestation of RA when the patient is overtaken by pain and swelling in a number of joints, accompanied by fever, loss of appetite and weight loss almost overnight.

This confusing pattern of initial symptoms has one common characteristic that usually distinguishes it from osteoarthritis or from the sort of aches and pains that follow exercise or muscle strain: in almost three-quarters of cases the pain or swelling is symmetrical: that is, both wrists, both ankles, both knees are affected.

Because it is rare for RA to present in an asymmetrical pattern of joints, a nurse or doctor first seeing a patient with such symptoms may be reluctant to make a diagnosis of RA. With time a typical symmetry of affected joints usually emerges.

Beth's story
Beth was 18 when she felt the first symptoms of RA (in the 1980s).

'I was at college studying the 'cello, doing drama classes with all sorts of athletic activity. I knew at once what the stiffness in my fingers and my shoulders meant. Our family doctor said he couldn't see any difference, but I knew. But because my mother had had severe RA for many years he sent me to a specialist. They started me on 12 aspirin a day straight away. I knew my 'cello-playing days were over.'

The natural history of RA

The term 'natural' history describes the course of an untreated illness. For example, if you catch a cold its natural history predicts that it will inhabit the various linings of your nose and throat, causing inflammation, coughing, sneezing and streaming, and will then clear up of its own accord after three to four days. In this context drugs or other medical interventions are 'unnatural'. These days most cases of RA are certainly not allowed to run their 'natural' course. Nevertheless it is important to chart the possible/probable natural course of a disease as a benchmark against which to measure the success of treatment and the best time to intervene.

RA may follow four different roads (see Figure 4). These routes were plotted before currently available medicines and therapeutic strategies that alter the course of the disease had been developed.

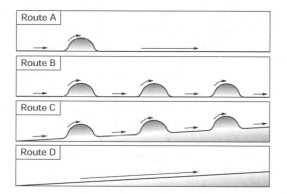

Figure 4   Untreated rheumatoid arthritis:
possible routes of progression

Route A

A single hummock like a sleeping policeman in the road. The road before and beyond is level. This course is known as spontaneous *remission* – the disease stops of its own accord. The common cold always ends with spontaneous remission; so do most cases of influenza. You can treat the symptoms, but the illness runs its course regardless and ultimately gives up and goes away.

To count as remission the RA must clearly have been there in the first place. During the 'bump' this will have been confirmed by positive responses to various blood tests described later in Chapter 4.

During remission these tests often return to normal. The symptoms abate and the patient will probably have taken little more than available over-the-counter pain-killers like aspirin or one of the non-steroid anti-inflammatory drugs (NSAIDs). Pain-killing treatment is looked at in detail in Chapter 7.

The good news is that about 20 per cent of patients experience spontaneous remission in RA. The bad news is that at least half of these relapse later – another sleeping policeman in the road. That leaves at most 10 per cent travelling along Route A.

Route B

This is a series of bumps in the road like a really emphatic traffic-calming system close to a primary school, but the road in between the bumps is flat. It's called 'remitting' because the remission is not total but repeated. The RA flares up, but in between the patient's health and joints return to normal. Provided that the flare-ups are not too close together and the movement of the joints is not permanently restricted, it is quite usual to treat people following this course with pain-killing drugs only when they are affected. But if the bumps come close together, or are prolonged so that the patient's life is disrupted, or if there are clear signs that the affected joints are suffering permanent damage, then the doctors may decide to try something that can alter the course of the disease, without actually curing it. These drugs are called 'disease-modifying anti-rheumatic drugs' (DMARDs) and are most effective if used early on in the course of RA before damage to the affected joints is severe enough to show up on X-ray. These drugs are looked at in detail in Chapter 8.

Route C

Here the traffic-calming system is on an up-hill slope. The course of RA is 'remitting progressive': it comes and goes, but after each episode the patient does not revert to normal health. Inflammation is probably still present in the joints between acute attacks and they may sustain lasting damage. The patient's daily life will become progressively more restricted. If the RA is going down this road doctors will almost certainly prescribe DMARDs.

Route D

There are no bumps on this road, just a steady up-hill climb. This is the 'progressive' course of RA. Usually the progression is gradual, with joint damage and loss of mobility happening slowly over time and the pain and swelling reduced by pain-killing drugs. Nevertheless, if the patient is following this route doctors will almost certainly decide to start treatment with DMARDs early, with the goal of halting the damage caused by unremitting inflammation.

Anna's story

When she was in her early forties Anna noticed her fingers feeling stiff and uncomfortable. 'I'm a keen dressmaker. It was gradually becoming clear to me that doing anything fiddly with a needle was well-nigh impossible.' At first Anna thought she was starting osteoarthritis. She took cod-liver oil capsules and told herself that things would soon clear up. But they didn't. One morning her joints felt so unbelievably stiff she didn't want to get out of bed. Her husband persuaded her to see her GP.

The GP took some blood from Anna's arm and sent it off for tests. She asked a lot of questions, during the course of which Anna remembered that something like this had happened years before: excruciatingly painful fingers in both hands making it almost impossible for her to sew or even turn on a tap. That time her husband had been abroad and Anna had soldiered on, taking aspirin and hoping things would clear up as they eventually did. Anna's GP suspected that Anna had started out on Route A of RA (remission) but was now embarking on Route B – remitting. Sure enough, when the tests came back RA was confirmed. Anna and her doctor discussed the options. They decided Anna would take just NSAIDs for the pain and inflammation for the time being, but that if the symptoms were no better in three weeks, the GP would prescribe one of the DMARDs to prevent permanent damage to Anna's joints.

How does treatment alter the course of RA?

The doctors' quandary

The variable and uncertain routes taken in RA stymie the doctors treating it as much as the patient. Should they throw the armoury of powerful drugs at the condition early on, or should they wait?

A patient is confirmed with an acute attack of RA. Is she

embarking upon Route A, B C or D? A spontaneous remission (Route A) is a two in ten possibility; they could simply treat the pain and reduce inflammation with an NSAID and cross fingers for remission, or they could forge ahead with more radical treatments that offer the hope of warding off the long-term damage caused by inflammation, which seem to work best if used early in the disease.

But the choice is not even as simple as that. Drugs have side effects. Even routine pain-killers produce *some* side effects for *some* patients, and the more radical treatments have the potential to cause more and more severe ones – again, it must be emphasized, in *some* patients. Broadly speaking, the more powerful the drug the greater the risk of side effects. So against the value of prescribing early on there is therefore a powerful argument for holding back the big guns until the medical team is sure that without them things are definitely getting worse.

Even then the path is not straightforward. If they decide to prescribe second-line drugs, which do they go for? These days the doctors are spoilt for choice. In addition to chemically based drugs that come under heading of DMARDs there are drugs that modify the inflammatory process biologically. (More about these biological response modifiers in Chapter 9.) But out of this impressive arsenal of drugs no one can predict which drug will work for which patient. Inevitably it turns out to be a question of trial and error. (See Box 4 opposite, 'Matching drugs to individual patients'.)

How is treatment different from cure?

In the days before modern antibiotics were discovered (before the Second World War), someone who developed cystitis (a common bacterial infection that causes inflammation of the bladder) would be given an old tried-and-tested medicine known as Mist Pot Cit – pharmacists' shorthand for a solution (mist) of potassium citrate. This treated the worst symptom of cystitis – burning urine – by turning it from acid to alkaline. This medicine didn't cure cystitis, it just made it less uncomfortable, and eventually the bacteria causing it gave up and went home.

Today doctors prescribe antibiotics for cystitis and it usually disappears – is cured – completely within days. That's the difference between treatment and cure.

Most chronic conditions like RA cannot be cured at the moment.

Box 4   *Matching drugs to individual patients*

The difficulty of finding out which drug works for which patient is not unique to RA. The vast majority of drugs – with the possible exception of antibiotics and anaesthetics – affect patients variably. That is because patients have subtle variations in their genetic make-up that make some of them click with a drug while others get side effects but no benefit.

The mapping of the human genome – the grand project that will eventually tell us what genes we have, what their role is, and which ones vary slightly from person to person making us subtly different from each other, while still recognizably human – will eventually answer this question.

Some of these small genetic variations have already been discovered. We know that one makes some women more prone to breast cancer, and that there are others that make people more vulnerable to certain infectious diseases. Studies are going on into links between genes and asthma, Alzheimer's disease and many other conditions that also depend upon environmental triggers, like RA. Scientists believe that research will eventually reveal which genetic variations make people responsive to one drug or another and which make them susceptible to which side effect. Then the goal of 'tailor-made' drugs which work for all the appropriate group of patients will be achievable.

Until then doctors have to rely on trial and error plus educated guesswork.

This is true for a large number of conditions – coronary artery disease, diabetes, asthma – some of which we may one day be able to cure. Others which are a part of natural ageing are less likely to be curable. With chronic diseases doctors are happy to be able to reduce symptoms and prolong remission. Remission, however, is not the same as cure.

The vast majority of people with RA can continue their normal way of life with only minimal modifications thanks to modern treatment, which includes a lot more than drugs. But, as it is for those who have had cancer, the disease continues to be a shadow in the background even when they are in remission. There is always the risk of recurrence. No one is absolutely cured.

This, of course, may change if and when improved understanding of what has gone wrong in RA leads to better, more precise drugs to correct it.

What happens if RA becomes worse?

It would be dishonest to suggest that modern therapy can make everything in the RA garden lovely. This is a serious disease. It can have unpleasant and permanent consequences. What starts in one set of joints (on both sides of the body), for example the hands and wrists, is quite likely to spread to other joints, the ankles and feet. If the inflammation persists joints may become deformed, bones may even fuse (join together), other parts of the body may be affected: tendons, blood vessels, the lungs. It is an unpredictable course. However, significant pain and disability in the one set of joints does not mean that it will automatically be as disabling and uncomfortable if it affects other joints.

How severe can disability be?

In the past, people with RA quite often ended up in a wheel-chair or housebound like Beth's mother, finding it very difficult to move about or do anything requiring strength and agility with their hands. It was a really bad story, and many of those with these bad stories are still around. Many people may have seen a poor old grandma or great-aunt with hands quite unrecognizably deformed with RA.

Since the 1990s new drugs and new ways of using them have made a real difference. But DMARDs have only come into use gradually over fifty years, so that older RA sufferers have not benefited from them for very long. In addition doctors take a much more pro-active attitude to RA these days. They intervene sooner with more effective drugs that prevent some of the worst manifestations of RA.

That said, even today there is a small minority of people whose RA is so severe that it makes them seriously ill and inflicts major disability.

For about 5 per cent of sufferers RA is a life-threatening condition. More about this group and what doctors can do for them is discussed in Chapter 12.

4

Diagnosing RA: a testing time

Shirley's story
Shirley was nearly 50 and the uncomplaining sort. She only went to her doctor when the pain in her hands made it so difficult for her to turn the steering wheel that she almost collided with another car. She hated to bother the doctor, she said; the doctor was such a busy man. And, yes, the doctor was busy and to begin with he thought it was just osteoarthritis and recommended aspirin. It was nearly two months before Shirley's husband got her back to the surgery. The swelling and stiffness were so bad she had given up driving, and now her ankles and feet were affected as well. Rather late, the GP suspected that she had RA. He sent a blood sample for tests and his suspicions were confirmed: they found RF. Worried about the delay, he prescribed NSAIDs for Shirley and decided to get her an appointment with a specialist. The waiting time in their area was five months.

The danger of delay

Unpalatable fact number one: three-quarters of those with early RA are likely to develop joint erosion – that's permanent damage to the joints – within two years from the start of symptoms. Unpalatable fact number two: half of those with unremitting RA have usually stopped work ten years from diagnosis. Early diagnosis and early treatment are vital.

The causes of delay are several. First there is delay in consulting a doctor – 'It's just aches and pains. It'll soon get better. The doctor's so busy.' Second, GPs may not correctly identify the condition. They see hundreds of people with osteoarthritis, but only a handful with RA, and RA is treacherously deceptive. Third, even when the GP is on the ball, when tests confirm the diagnosis, it may still take months to get a patient an appointment with a specialist rheumatology department. In cases when RA does not respond to front-line anti-inflammatory drugs like NSAIDs the GP must choose between hounding the hospital for a specialist appointment and starting the patient on DMARDs in the practice.

Professor Paul Emery is head of rheumatology and rehabilitation research at the University of Leeds in the UK, and is Chair of the Collaboration to Assess and Refer Early (CARE) initiative. He said,

There is a definite need for physicians to identify RA early since we know the greatest amount of structural damage occurs within the first two years of disease onset, leading to disability. Early referral to a rheumatologist within the first 12 weeks of onset of symptoms, and treatment with a disease-modifying anti-rheumatic drug (DMARD) improve long-term outcomes for patients.

This is easier said than done.

The doctor's dilemma

Rheumatoid arthritis is a headache for the GP as well as the patient. There is no classic way to recognize RA sufferers as they come through the surgery door. There is no single definitive test that will reveal it. They come in with the most terrible pain, stiffness and swelling in their joints. Arthritis, yes, but what kind? They may say they feel generally off colour or show signs of fever; the joint pain may be mentioned but as an afterthought. Most patients think aches and pains are not important enough to bother a doctor with routinely. So the GP will try to narrow the field by ruling out other possible causes. It's called making a differential diagnosis. Even then certainty may elude her; many of the symptoms of RA are shared with one or another form of arthritis. But as all these unknowns hold her back, one certainty drives her forward: if it is RA it should not be left untreated.

Faced with the dilemma of unspecified joint pain, the GP's first step will be to take a detailed history and make a thorough assessment of the patient's physical symptoms. In this the doctor will be assisted by 'clinical guidelines' – basically tick-boxes for symptoms that the experts have discovered make a diagnosis of RA likely or probable.

Professor Emery's CARE initiative, putting the emphasis on getting RA patients to a rheumatoid specialist as soon as possible, says patients should be referred if any of the following is present:

- three or more swollen joints;
- particular hand joints swollen when the doctor checks with a 'squeeze test';
- morning stiffness lasting for half an hour or longer.

The American College of Rheumatology supplies a longer list of symptoms and suggests that four out of seven should be present to confirm a diagnosis:

1 morning stiffness in and around joints, lasting more than an hour;
2 arthritis of three or more joint areas involved simultaneously;
3 arthritis in at least one area of the wrist, or the small joints of the hand;
4 symmetrical joint involvement;
5 the presence of rheumatoid *nodules* (for a description of nodules see Chapter 5);
6 RF in the blood;
7 changes to the hand or wrist characteristic of RA visible on X-ray.

The reason the American College of Rheumatology list is longer than the UK CARE initiative's is that its diagnostic tests include those not done in the average GP's surgery in the UK. They have to be carried out at a hospital laboratory.

Drawing blood

But whether in a specialist department or a GP's surgery, the first steps to a diagnosis of RA are the same, and include drawing blood. After the history and the physical assessment, either the doctor or the practice nurse will take a sample of blood from the patient in order that it may be sent to the laboratory and analysed.

The blood is the transport system of the body. A great deal of information can be obtained by unpacking some of the things carried around the body in the bloodstream at any one time. Other bodily functions are also informative: urine, the fluid inside joints or the spine, blood-pressure readings and recordings of the electrical activity of the heart and brain. But with RA blood tests are vital, so you cannot afford to be squeamish about blood or needles. Resign yourself to having a lot of needles stuck into you – into veins to take blood, into the joint itself to take samples of synovial fluid and, at some stage, to inject things into the blood or the joint. (See Box 5 if this gives you the shivers.)

The first tests done on the patient's blood have a common objective: to determine whether the arthritis is caused by inflammation, and if it is, to try and discover what kind of inflammation. Even when the results come through, a cast-iron diagnosis will almost certainly not be available at this stage. But the GP will have narrowed the options and will know enough to be able to start treatment while referring the possible cases of RA to a specialist rheumatology department.

Early on four blood tests are routinely done to test for RA.

Box 5 *An abnormal fear of needles*

The scene is familiar: Woody Allen does it in the film *Sleeper*, and it's Hugh Grant's turn in *Nine Months*. They pass out at the sight of the hypodermic syringe. And apparently they are not unusual. An abnormal fear of needles or any other sharp object that threatens to penetrate the skin is officially recognized in the Diagnostic and Statistical Manual, fourth edition (DSM-IV), the psychiatrists' bible. It's called *Aichmophobia* or *Belonephobia* – the word *phobia* being Greek for 'fear'.

Researchers estimate that between 7 and 22 per cent of people may suffer from an abnormal fear of needles. They are mostly invisible and unmeasured because they go to incredible lengths in order to avoid having injections or giving blood. If untreated, squeamishness about needles gets in the way of much good medicine: immunizations against disease, blood transfusions, having an anaesthetic before surgery, not to mention pain-free dentistry. Some people's lives depend on needles: insulin for insulin-dependent diabetics can only be delivered by injection, and some people with multiple sclerosis need weekly shots of life-saving drugs.

Fear of needles may be acquired, through a nasty experience, or inborn – scientists can't agree – but it seems to run in families. One expert believes there may be a sound historic reason for the

---

- **Erythrocyte Sedimentation Rate (ESR)** This simple non-specific test measures the time it takes for the red blood cells (erythrocyte is Greek for 'red cell') in unclotted blood to form sediment at the bottom of a test-tube. If there is inflammation or there are auto-immune cells active in the body the sediment collects more rapidly. Further down the line the ESR is useful for monitoring the success of treatment because it slows down if the drugs the patient is taking are reducing inflammation. Its limitation is that sedimentation may speed up for all sorts of reasons: because the patient has an infection or from an inflammatory condition other than RA. And it slows down if the patient is taking certain common drugs, like penicillin, diuretics or vitamin A. But a doctor who has taken a thorough history will be alerted to this complication.

---

fear. In the past, fatal damage or death was often caused by sharp things – teeth, claws, fangs and tusks, or weapons like knives, spears, swords and arrows.

And for the needle-phobe the fear is not just psychological, it is measurably physiological. The sight, mention even, of a needle causes the blood pressure to drop and the heart-rate to slow. Insufficient blood reaches the brain; they turn pale, feel dizzy and sometimes pass out, like Hugh Grant.

Other researchers think that fainting could be compared to the way some animals play dead when faced with a predator or other threat. Collapsing on the surgery floor could be the human equivalent.

Whatever the cause or explanation, if you have RA you need to steel yourself to the needle, so to speak. On the internet there are numerous offers to cure phobias of every sort. Many involve hypnotherapy, but there are also a number of psychological techniques. Some, like desensitization, involve the gradual approach and acquired tolerance of the feared needle. Others, like neuro-linguistic programming, time line therapy or emotional freedom techniques, claim to work without exposing the phobic to the feared object and even to work over the telephone! (Details in Useful addresses at the end of the book.)

- **Rheumatoid factor (RF)** RF is one of the antibodies thought to be responsible for tissue damage in RA. You might think that finding an antibody with this name in the blood was proof positive that someone had RA. Would that it were so. Although it is found in the blood of at least 80 per cent of RA patients, and in higher concentrations the more severe the disease, it does not always show up at the early stages of RA. If the first test is negative the patient will be tested again at a later date. Occasionally RF is found in the blood of people with other forms of arthritis like lupus (SLE) or even other diseases: tuberculosis, malaria or hepatitis C. It is also naturally high in about 5 per cent of elderly people. However, in these cases the amount is usually lower than it is in people with RA. The amount of RF is expressed as a *titre,* a measure of quantity. RF in the blood of someone without the symptoms of RA may indicate that it will develop later in life.
- **C-reactive protein (CRP)** Like ESR, the presence of CRP is an indicator of acute inflammation, though not specifically RA. It is more sensitive than ESR because it is only rarely found in the blood of healthy people. CRP is produced by the liver in response to inflammation. High levels in the blood back up the evidence of the other two blood tests, and when it comes to monitoring treatment, lowered levels of CRP demonstrate success in reducing inflammation and the harm it can do.
- **CCP antibodies** Another blood test highly suggestive of RA is the presence of an antibody to a protein called CCP. If positive this hardens the diagnosis considerably because CCP antibodies are almost never found in the blood of someone without RA, although 40 per cent of sufferers may *not* have them. In medical terms this makes the test highly specific (only found in those with RA) but not sensitive (but not in everyone with RA). It has recently been discovered that, as with RF, those extremely rare individuals who have CCP antibodies but no evident RA may go on to develop it later in life.

Diagnostic tests carried out in hospital

While waiting for the test results a GP will probably prescribe NSAIDs (see Chapter 7) to relieve pain and reduce inflammation because they have relatively few side effects.

When the results of preliminary blood tests confirm the GP's tentative diagnosis, if not before, she will almost certainly refer the patient to out-patients at a specialist rheumatology department where more sophisticated tests and treatment can be undertaken.

A rheumatologist will probably sample the synovial fluid in one of the affected joints, and take X-rays.

- **Synovial fluid** Unsurprising in view of the fact that it is the place where the trouble starts, additional information can be gathered from taking a sample of joint fluid. This tricky procedure requires very precise positioning of a needle to *aspirate* (suck up) a sample of fluid from inside the joint. If increased numbers of neutrophils are discovered the diagnosis of inflammatory arthritis is confirmed. An analysis of synovial fluid can rule out other forms of arthritis like gout caused by crystals forming in the joint. The rheumatoid specialist can also check whether an infection could be the cause of inflammation. This is especially important if the patient presents with a fever, or has exceptional tenderness, swelling or warmth in a single joint.
- **X-ray images** In the early stages of RA these may be less helpful than when the condition has advanced and prolonged inflammation has caused actual tissue damage. Nevertheless, X-rays taken early on can provide a useful yard-stick against which the progress of the disease and its treatment may be measured. Rheumatologists look for early signs of bone thinning, and if the condition progresses X-rays may reveal tiny holes in the bone beneath the damaged cartilage – *erosion* – and a narrowing of the space in the joint caused by loss of cartilage. At this stage the diagnosis of RA has finally become conclusive.

And, for the majority of RA patients, this is probably the full extent of diagnostic procedures they will have to endure. The same tests will be repeated in the course of monitoring the progress of the disease and the success or otherwise of treatment, and some others may be necessary to check the side effects of some of the powerful drugs that are part of treatment. We will discuss these in the chapters on drug treatment.

But for a small group of patients with suspected RA these routine diagnostic tests may not lead to an unequivocal diagnosis. In these cases the rheumatologist may decide he needs to examine the actual joint lining – the synovium – where the early changes caused by inflammation in RA take place.

The rheumatologist may take a *biopsy* – a tiny sample of living tissue withdrawn by means of a special needle inserted into the joint, which may then be tested and examined under a microscope in the laboratory. This is done in out-patients, under local anaesthetic, and causes some people mild discomfort. Alternatively the specialist may prefer to examine the interior of the joint visually before taking a sample. This is called *arthroscopic* biopsy – a 'scope' being a fibre-optic probe that provides an image of various internal organs, in this case a joint (*arthro*). This is done in an operating theatre under local, partial or general anaesthetic. The probe, which is about the thickness of a pencil, is inserted into the joint so that it can be viewed and a sample of tissue taken for laboratory analysis.

Occasionally biopsies of other organs – muscle, lung, nerve or skin – may need to be taken. As we have explained, RA is a systemic disease: the joints may be most severely affected, but the whole body is involved to some extent; more of such complications in the next chapter.

Anthea's story
Anthea first suffered fleeting joint pains in her early twenties. She was studying to be a nurse and often had a lot of strenuous physical work to do, so at first she put it down to muscle strain. But her professional training alerted her to the fact that when the same joints in both her hands became stiff and painful it was one of the classic signs of RA. She had been tired and generally unwell for some time so she went to her family doctor and asked for tests to be done. They were all negative: no RF, no notable increase in ESR; no CPC. 'My doctor told me it was all in my mind. I was over-tired and nurses always thought they had every disease under the sun.' Anthea took pain-killers and tried to ignore the agony in her hands first thing in the morning before the drugs took effect. Fortunately she told her story to one of her colleagues in the hospital, and, without a referral, a specialist rheumatologist looked at her joints. More tests, and still no RF, but this time slightly increased ESR and CPC. He was concerned enough to do an arthroscopic biopsy and confirmed the early signs of RA damage to the cartilage. He prescribed DMARDs straight away in the hope of preventing further damage. This was nearly three years after Anthea had first reported her symptoms.

5
Symptoms of RA outside the joints

Fatigue plus ...

As we have explained, RA is a systemic disease: that is to say, it affects the whole system although the primary attack is against the synovial joints. The medical term for such symptoms – some common, others rare – is *extra-articular*, meaning 'outside the joint'.

The most common extra-articular symptom suffered by people with RA is a generalized sense of being ill: fatigue, loss of appetite, aches and pains and low-grade fever, a pattern most of us associate with having some kind of infection. One person described it colourfully as 'It's as if my body were a battleground.' And in some ways it is. The auto-immune system is up in arms, releasing the firepower of inflammation. But in the case of RA the enemy is within. It's fighting part of your own body. The system is at war. For many people this malaise is minor discomfort they are able to ignore, though in some cases glands in the neck, armpit and groin – the *lymph nodes* – may become swollen, an indication that inflammation is at work all over the body. With the exception of the latter, the condition is so like other less serious forms of illness that it is often not identified as connected with the swollen, painful joints which are the hallmark of arthritis.

People with a history of anxiety and depression are more likely to suffer from debilitating fatigue with RA than others.

Dorothy's story
Dorothy was well known to her doctor. She had suffered from bouts of depression since the 1970s. When her children were still young she had become addicted to the popular tranquillizer Valium, and 20 years later she had gone through a bad menopause. Keeping Dorothy on an even keel taxed the GP's patience and ingenuity. When Dorothy called him out because she felt so ill she had been unable to get out of bed for two days, he started running through in his mind which antidepressant he could possibly prescribe that would do no harm. But when he came to examine her, he discovered that the joints of her hands, wrists and

37

feet were stiff and swollen on both sides of her body. He took blood, and when the results of the tests came back from the laboratory his suspicion that she had developed RA was confirmed. Dorothy's painful joints responded well to drug treatment, NSAIDs followed later by DMARDs, and within six months she had recovered most of the movement in her hands and feet. Over the next 11 years she had two further acute episodes of RA and they were both preceded by same severe and debilitating fatigue.

Disorders of the blood

Another common extra-articular symptom of RA which contributes to the tiredness and malaise is *anaemia*, a condition in which the number of red cells in the blood – the ones that carry oxygen around the body – decreases as a result of long-standing inflammation. Some 50–70 per cent of RA sufferers may develop anaemia if their RA remains untreated, which is one of the reasons why carrying out a full blood analysis is so important during diagnosis. Anaemia usually improves once inflammation is brought under control, but if it doesn't a drug that stimulates the production of red blood cells can be prescribed if, for example, the patient has to undergo surgery and risks losing blood.

Another kind of anaemia sometimes develops as a result of the drugs that are prescribed to treat the inflammation in RA. In some people NSAIDs irritate the lining of the stomach and increase the amount of blood loss that occurs naturally into the gut. If this happens the offending drugs may be temporarily withdrawn while something to heal the gut lining is taken.

There are a lot of fortunately less common complications in RA. Box 6 opposite describes one of these, Felty's syndrome.

Skin complications

About 25 per cent of RA sufferers develop small (up to 5 centimetre) nodules under the skin. Rheumatoid nodules are more common in men and usually occur in those who also have rheumatoid factor in their blood. Like RF they are regarded as confirming the diagnosis, but they usually appear some time after the onset of the disease.

Box 6   *A rare complication: Felty's syndrome*

Felty's syndrome is a rare blood disorder which results in an enlarged spleen and a decreased white cell count in addition to anaemia. This loss of white cells, part of the body's natural defence system, means that the patient becomes more vulnerable to infection. The number of platelets – part of the blood-clotting mechanism – may also diminish (*thrombocytopenia*; thrombo-cyte means clotting cell), increasing the risk of excessive bleeding. Less than 1 per cent of RA sufferers develop this condition, and usually only after having had RA for many years. A number of drugs may correct it, or if all else fails the spleen can be surgically removed.

Just to confuse things, while Felty's syndrome and a low platelet count is extremely rare, it is quite common for people with RA to have an increased platelet count (thrombocytosis). This is relatively harmless and is usually corrected when the arthritis is treated.

Nodules don't hurt, unless they are somewhere they get knocked or have pressure applied to them, like the back of the heel where a shoe presses, and are otherwise harmless though aesthetically unpleasing. They appear close to affected joints, where the skin is stretched, in particular the elbow and upper forearm or Achilles tendon at the back of the ankle, and they may come and go following the pattern of the disease.

Microscopic inspection of the cells that make up a nodule suggests that they may start with small blood vessels (capillaries) becoming inflamed and broken, another complication of RA. It is possible to shrink them, by the local injection of anti-inflammatory drugs, or they may be surgically removed, but they tend to recur.

Very occasionally rheumatoid nodules develop in other organs – the lungs, eyes, heart or vocal cords – but even here they rarely cause serious problems.

Problems with the eyes and mouth

Inflammation can strike all over the body, and about 15 per cent of those with RA find it affects the glands that produce tears and saliva so that they end up with uncomfortably dry eyes and mouth. This is known as *sicca syndrome* – sicca meaning dry – but when the damage to the glands is caused by rheumatoid inflammation the condition is also sometimes called Sjögren's syndrome, after the physician who first described it. As anyone who has suffered from a blocked tear-duct knows, tears are not just for weeping or responding to peeled onions, they lubricate the movement of the eye and eyelids and provide protection from wind or bright light. If eyes are not constantly bathed with tears they can become very itchy and sore, as can the eyelids. The same goes for insufficient saliva; food turns to ash in your mouth. Both problems which can start with rheumatoid inflammation of the glands producing the fluid can also be aggravated by some medication.

There is a treatment for dry eyes called 'artificial tears'. Anyone suffering excessive dryness in the eye with pain or redness should always inform their doctor because other, rarer conditions that affect other parts of the eye can be more serious.

Problems with tendons, blood vessels, lungs and heart

The scatter-gun of inflammation strikes all over the body but is more likely to hit connective tissues which are closely related to the synovial joint lining, the first casualty of RA. Tendons, for example those in the heel, elbow or wrist, are lined with a similar membrane and may become inflamed. In the wrist, swollen tendons can compress a nerve at the point where it passes into the hand, causing burning or tingling in the palm and numbness and pain in the middle fingers. This condition is known as *carpal tunnel* syndrome after the channel in the wrist where the compression occurs. It may also be caused by a wrist fracture or from some repetitive wrist or finger movement like typing, sewing or using an electric drill. Again, once the RA is treated these problems usually subside.

Helen's story
Helen arrived at her doctor's asking for sleeping pills. The GP, who had diagnosed Helen's RA some years previously, knew Helen had experienced a series of flare-ups although the DMARD that had been prescribed for her appeared to have brought the

major problems in her wrists and fingers under control. Rather than writing a quick 'scrip' the GP probed Helen for why she thought she needed sleeping pills. 'It's my hands,' she explained, 'I keep waking at night with this terrible numbness in my fingers, and tingling in my hands. Then I start to worry about whether I will have to stop work, and I just can't get back to sleep.' When the GP enquired further it turned out the numbness chiefly affected the three middle fingers of Helen's hands. She also explained that her work in a busy estate agent's office involved typing up the details of the properties that came on to their books. She had had problems with her hands during the day as well. The doctor diagnosed carpal tunnel syndrome as result of inflamed tendons in Helen's wrists. She suggested that Helen could try wearing a splint on her wrists at night or alternatively have an injection of a corticosteroid directly into the site of the inflammation. This is a highly skilled operation not every GP will undertake personally, but Helen's GP had had sufficient experience to do it for her. The numbness was relieved. She began sleeping all night again, and without sleeping pills.

Inflammation is more serious when it affects blood vessels. This is called *vasculitis* and is fortunately rare; it is seen mostly in people who also have high levels of RF in their blood. What seems to happen is that the excessive number of antibodies produced in the blood by plasma cells (see Chapter 2) clump together and then cling to the vessel wall, causing inflammation. The seriousness of vasculitis depends on the location of the blood vessels affected. If they are in the skin ulcers may develop or tiny characteristic 'splinter' lesions around and under the finger-nails. These are easily treated with careful washing in mild antiseptic and the application of a sterile dressing. Vasculitis is more serious if it affects blood vessels leading to nerves, when localized numbness or weakness may develop. In this instance, short-term treatment with strong anti-inflammatory drugs called *corticosteroids* may be necessary. (Corticosteroids are discussed in Chapter 8.)

Between 10 and 20 per cent of those with RA at some stage develop *pleurisy*, inflammation of the pleura, the membrane lining the lung. This causes pain deep in the chest with breathing. Occasionally there is also a build-up of fluid in the pleural cavity which it is necessary to drain with a special needle (an out-patient procedure). Corticosteroid drugs may be required for this complication, because without specific treatment there is always the risk that pleurisy can lead to inflammation of the lungs themselves – *pneumonia* – a potentially fatal illness.

Another cause of pain in breathing occurs when the collar- or chest-bones (the *clavicles* and *sternum*) develop arthritis. (The sternoclavicular joints are marked in Figure 1 on p. 11.) This is experienced by about 30 per cent of those with RA and, like most of these complications, disappears when the inflammation is brought under control.

Very occasionally rheumatoid nodules similar to those in the skin develop in the lung. They usually cause no symptoms, but if they are detected on an X-ray the doctors will usually take a sample with a biopsy just to reassure themselves that it is not a more serious kind of growth.

The heart also has a membrane lining, the *pericardium*, which may become inflamed in RA. This is called *pericarditis* and is relatively common – up to 40 per cent of sufferers may experience it. It often causes no symptoms at all, but doctors detect the tell-tale sounds of fluid when they listen to the patient's heart or it may show up on X-ray. If the patient does feel something, it is likely to be chest pain and possibly breathlessness. Pericarditis usually responds to corticosteroids, and the build-up of fluid is rarely so great that it has to be drained. The heart itself is hardly ever involved in RA.

Problems with bone

In Chapter 2 (Box 2, p. 14) we provided a brief introduction to bone cells – osteoblasts (bone-creating) and osteoclasts (bone-absorbing) – whose activity becomes unbalanced in RA. The osteoclasts get overactive compared with the cells that replace lost bone. Recent research has implicated a group of pro-inflammatory cytokines (cell messengers, see Chapter 2) in this process. They produce a substance that stimulates the osteoclasts. This also happens during the menopause and the result in both cases is a loss of bone density known as *osteoporosis,* the 'thinning' of bone. It means bones break more easily and has been known to be a major health problem for a sizable proportion of old people, particularly women, for many years. In the past it was difficult to measure. As an Australian researcher once said: 'You can't very well go round throwing old ladies down stairs.' But a new technique called *densitometry* has made it possible to test the density of bone without breaking it.

Osteoporosis is more of a problem for women (with or without RA), partly because they generally have lower bone mass than men to start with. Men with RA do not entirely escape the complication because they occasionally have low levels of the hormone testosterone, which causes additional bone loss. There are also a range of life-style factors – smoking, not taking enough exercise, or not having enough calcium and vitamin D in the diet – that make osteoporosis more likely. (A study suggests that a diet rich in calcium and vitamin D makes elderly women less likely to develop RA.)

And the double whammy is that the very corticosteroids that come to the rescue in some of the acute extra-articular complications of RA like vasculitis or pleurisy can in themselves make bone loss worse.

These extra-articular symptoms make depressing reading. Take comfort from the fact that many are comparatively rare; others, like nodules, though common are inconvenient rather than really troublesome. All either subside when the RA is treated or are susceptible to specific medication.

Part 2: Treating and beating RA

6

Rest and rehabilitation for inflamed joints

When writing about a complex illness it is difficult not to treat the subject primarily as medical science. As we try to explain the anatomy of human joints, how the immune system works (and goes wrong) or diagnostic tests that pick up clues as to where things are going wrong, the most important thing of all inevitably gets pushed to one side: the experience of the patient. This means *your* experience.

Coping with RA is the core of this book. All the medical science in the world cannot overcome the painful business of being ill. But understanding, while it may not cure, can modify that experience for the better, rather like the drugs prescribed for RA. Grasp the underlying process of the disease and you can take charge of it rather than letting it flatten you. And the best treatment and coping strategies are guided by scientific knowledge. We have done our best to explain RA. Now we come to the main theme: what can you, your medical team and your nearest and dearest do about it?

It's unavoidable that in dealing with treatment there will be a lot about drugs, and some pretty sophisticated ones at that. (We tackle these in Chapters 7, 8 and 9.) But we will start with some things you can do yourself, at home – by adopting important, constructive physical activities. Later, in Chapter 11, we discuss dealing with emotions, and in Chapter 12 modifying your life-style. Self-help is the key to overcoming the negative feelings that come in the wake of chronic, painful disease. (See Box 7 overleaf.)

Box 7   *Self-help really works*

Studies in the USA of people who followed the Arthritis Founda-tion's Self-help Course found they suffered 20 per cent less pain and made 40 per cent fewer visits to their doctor than other people with RA. The course is designed to enable people to understand the disease and to adopt an active role in managing it (very much the goals of this book). The Arthritis Foundation says that when people feel greater control over their disease it 'builds a sense of confidence in their ability to function and lead a full, active and independent life'.

How much should you rest?

As children we were often told that if you are feeling ill the best thing is to go to bed and rest. The pain and stiffness of RA is usually worse early in the morning. The most natural thing in the world is to feel like staying in bed. But you will also be advised to exercise and maximize the mobility of the affected joints. This is not as contradictory as it may at first seem. Rest and exercise work together and need to be finely balanced in RA; too much of either is probably a bad thing.

In recent years there has been a swing in medical opinion on the relationship between rest and exercise. Forty years ago lengthy bed-rest was flavour of the month. People were sometimes taken into hospital and kept in bed for months at a time. And since inflamed joints usually improve with rest, especially if they are also splinted to protect and support their immobility (see Chapter 12 for splints), the practice appeared to work.

But looked at long term, other parts of the body don't do so well under prolonged bed-rest. Unused muscles become weaker, bones lose calcium and become more brittle, physical fitness declines when the body is not put to use, and being in bed all day is not the most cheerful place to be: you certainly can't do much work or carry on your normal domestic routines from bed. The scene was set for a change of emphasis.

How athletic can you be with RA?

In the 1980s and 1990s doctors following a holistic, whole-person approach to disease management discovered that light exercise, while not damaging inflamed joints, was an aid to improved physical and emotional health. Exercise to maintain a joint's range of movement and to strengthen supporting muscle systems gradually became standard.

Everyone has become much more exercise-conscious in recent years. The value of regular *aerobic exercise* which builds up the resilience and capacity of the heart, lungs and circulation is now recognized as an integral part of healthy living. These values have affected attitudes towards exercise in the management of physical and mental illness. A number of therapists began to investigate whether people whose RA was under control could benefit from exercise that not only maintained the flexibility of their joints but increased physical strength and endurance. At the University of Missouri, Columbia, a physical therapist called Marion Minor reported encouraging results with advanced strengthening exercises and low-impact aerobic exercise for people with arthritis. They demonstrated improved stamina, less fatigue and an improved level of general physical functioning. They took less time off work and spent less time with their doctors.

As more rheumatology departments developed exercise programmes and put them into practice the benefits became widely recognized. Exercise not only improves the symptoms of RA – less pain, improved energy levels, physical strength, joint stability and general physical functioning – it also improves the patient's quality of life. This elusive commodity known to health professionals as a '*qualy*' is so prized that health departments and medical researchers now attempt to measure it by asking patients to answer tick-box questionnaires. Patients who take exercise tick the boxes for less breakable bones, less muscle tension, lower stress and anxiety levels, improved energy levels, increased self-esteem and a better night's sleep.

Lisa's story
Lisa, from Ohio in the USA, is a 35-year-old dietician. She was diagnosed with RA eight years ago. She was very active before her illness. She found tremendous support and information

47

through the US Arthritis Foundation and is now teaching a self-help class for them. She says, 'Before I got RA, I did a lot of running and in-line skating, but now the best exercises for me are non-impact or low-impact, such as speed walking, swimming, and bike riding (depending on how my wrists feel).'

An exercise programme for RA

An exercise programme designed to minimize the effect of a serious illness should naturally be planned as part of the overall medical scheme of things and with a trained physiotherapist. The exact approach favoured by individual therapists or rheumatology departments varies, and the account of exercise programmes in this chapter is not a substitute for professional guidance. The timing of exercise will be affected by the course of the illness, and the level of exercise undertaken by each patient has to be matched to their personal inclination and aptitude – not least whether they have been taking some form of regular exercise before becoming ill. Let's take a short tour round the kinds of exercise usually recommended and outline what they are intended to achieve.

At the most acute stages of RA, if you have fever and fatigue, bed-rest remains irresistible and recommended, provided you feel comfortable in bed. Even when the eye of the storm has passed, regular rest periods remain the order of the day. As with so many treatment programmes for chronic disease, the exact quantity of rest and exercise undertaken depends on the individual patient and the course of the disease, but in general little and often is better than long periods when it comes to lying down. Alternating exercise and rest is also recommended, possibly combining the two: lying down while doing gentle exercise like rotating the ankles and wrists, flexing the elbows and opening and shutting the hands, never overstepping the pain threshold, accompanied by deep breathing and calm, soothing thoughts, can be as relaxing as sleep.

Many people with RA find it helps to make minor modifications to their bed at home. To take the weight off painful feet and ankles a cradle that lifts the bedclothes from your lower limbs can be fitted. If you are to spend long periods in bed a board laid across the bottom half of the mattress will enable you to walk your feet back and forth under the cradle while lying down as gentle exercise. You could go one better than prone and lie on a slant-board. This aids the circulation as well as relieving the joints from the pressure of gravity.

Even at the acute stage of RA a regular exercise programme has an important role to play. The first kind of exercise described below plus a modest amount of muscle-strengthening exercise may be undertaken.

Range-of-motion exercise

These are probably the most crucial exercises for RA sufferers, especially when the joints are inflamed during a flare-up. (They're not a bad idea for someone with OA either.) The goal of range-of-motion exercises is to reduce stiffness and minimize loss of mobility in the affected joints. They take the joint through the fullest range of movement which it can manage once or twice a day or whenever you feel the need to reduce stiffness. Pay special attention to the point at which movement becomes difficult or impossible but don't push it to the point of pain. Once the acute inflammation has died down, range-of-motion exercises become part of the warm-up to the daily exercise routine. A pattern of ten minutes warm-up, fifteen minutes work-out, five minutes cool-down is common.

Stretching is a variation on range-of-motion exercise. It involves stretching the joint to *just beyond* the limit of comfort, as opposed to staying just within the comfort zone. No one will tell you to stretch to the level of actual pain and you shouldn't 'bounce' the joint in an attempt to extend it further. By putting the joint through its paces regularly, stiffness and pain are reduced. Range-of-motion exercises are even better done in water because the buoyancy of the water supports the body and protects the joints from rapid or stressful movement.

Exercise to strengthen muscles and joints

Muscles that have become weakened during acute inflammation need to be rebuilt by exercise. Muscle strength and tone matters, not only for general functionality but to support and protect joints. There is a chain reaction: inflammation, swelling and pain all affect the joints, causing tendons and ligaments to stretch, leading to the joints being less stable, and at the same time muscles become weaker through lack of use because of the pain and fail to support the damaged joint. Strengthening muscle with exercise can break this vicious circle.

Strengthening exercises come at different levels. *Isometric exercise* involves clenching and unclenching muscle groups without external movement. It can be done lying down and should be part of the exercise routine even when the joints are seriously inflamed to minimize the weakening of muscles from disuse. Isometric strengthening exercises introduce an external pressure point. They will usually be introduced once the acute inflammatory stage has died down. For example, you might push against the wall, tightening your arm muscles but without moving wrists, elbows or shoulders. This strengthens the muscles and protects the joints. Moving your joints against resistance – i.e. doing the same thing lying prone (push-ups) – is definitely out. Push-ups involve lifting the body's weight, and weights (with very few exceptions) do not form part of an RA exercise routine.

The final stage of isometric exercises involves pushing against an exercise band. These are commercially available or you can improvise using an elastic belt, bungee cords or a length of garden hose. This form of exercise is sometimes possible while the joints are still moderately inflamed and can definitely be attempted once the RA is under control and the inflammation has stabilized.

There is evidence that people with RA can become extremely fit using aerobic exercise. It increases stamina, reduces fatigue and pain and makes them more positive.

There is no evidence that aerobic exercise increases joint inflammation if carried out carefully, in stages under the supervision of a trained specialist, though exercise sometimes reveals that a joint you hadn't previously been aware of is inflamed.

Beth, always improvising in the care of her RA, recommends sitting and bouncing on one of those enlarged children's balls with ears. Sadly, she tells us, hers is currently out of action because the dog bit it.

Sharon's story
Sharon had been a keen amateur tennis player and when she was diagnosed with RA she was devastated. She stayed away from work and often couldn't drag herself out of bed in the morning. Getting her to her doctor and hospital appointments required

major effort on the part of her boyfriend, Karl. But he persisted. He read up everything he could get his hands on about living with RA and realized that unless she was prepared to be pro-active in coping with her illness, things could get worse. It was Karl who persuaded her to make an appointment with the physiotherapist, part of the team at the rheumatology department where she was being seen for her illness. The physiotherapist outlined a practical exercise regime for Sharon. She told her that there was every possibility that she would be able to play tennis again, though her overhead smash might not be quite as lethal. Twice a day Karl sat and did exercises with Sharon until gradually her confidence increased and the pain and stiffness began to ease. The inflammation was coming under control and her joints were assisted in their recovery by the fact that she had been physically fit before she got ill. Then one day Karl came home and found her in bed and in a deep depression again. She had taken out her racket and tried to do a few shots. 'The inflammation is back,' she wept, 'and now it's in my shoulders; I'll never be able to play tennis again.'

The physiotherapist was consulted; her RA had not flared up again. The shoulders had probably been slightly inflamed all along but Sharon had only become aware of it when trying to do over-arm strokes. 'You should only apply external pressure to your joints in very small doses,' she was advised. 'For the time being, stick to a gentle pat-ball if you must use your racket.'

Exercise for endurance

The heart is a pump made of muscle. Just as the muscles in your limbs become weak with disuse, so if the heart, lungs and blood vessels are not made to work at capacity regularly they also start to function under par. *Cardiovascular exercise* (the 'cardio' bit relates to the heart, 'vascular' refers to the blood vessels and lung function is also involved) is important for general fitness for everyone, especially as they grow older and spend less time on the sports field and longer in front of the telly. The role of cardiovascular exercise is to enable your body to perform over time without fatigue (endurance) and also to summon up spurts of greater energy when required – like running for a bus or playing tennis. This kind of exercise increases the capacity of the heart, lungs and blood vessels to work efficiently under stress by using oxygen efficiently. The word 'aerobic' implies making use of oxygen. The best kind of cardiovascular exercise for someone with RA will involve moderate effort but no jolting of joints (as in jumping – impact exercise), so swimming (breast-stroke rather than crawl if the shoulders are affected), walking, cycling, climbing up and down stairs (unless the knees are still inflamed). (Boxes 8, 9 (opposite) and 10 (p. 54) offer some tips.) Depending on the joints affected some form of low-impact aerobic exercise – like patting a ball against the wall or dancing (waltz, not salsa) – may also be attempted once the inflammation is in retreat. Once the muscles show signs of regaining strength and supporting affected joints adequately it may be possible to start working with weights, under professional guidance.

You have probably heard exercise fanatics talk about 'feeling the burn' or say, 'If you don't sweat it's no good.' This is because to improve your stamina cardiovascular performance you must increase your heart-rate (the number of beats your heart does each minute). If you have RA the sweating is not essential, but you will be aware of your pulse-rate increasing (the blood is being driven through your vessels at a faster rate) and you will probably be a bit breathless, at least to begin with. You are putting your heart through its paces and to do it good you should keep it up there for at least 15 minutes (ideally 30), and do it regularly three or four times a week. As you become fitter, exercise requires less effort and your pulse and heart-rate revert to normal quite quickly afterwards.

Once you have established a routine of half an hour's exercise several times a week you can vary the proportion of the exercises you do each time. You can reduce the amount of muscle-strengthening exercises as your muscles grow stronger and increase the time spent on cardiovascular endurance exercise. Range-of-motion exercises should be a permanent part of the routine for all affected joints. At all stages the exercise routine should be modified to allow for any joints that have become deformed by the RA.

Always remember, you are doing this to maintain fitness and compensate for the injury of an inflammatory disease. You are not in training for a Marathon. If you find yourself short of breath after exercise or experience prolonged fatigue, if you feel dizzy, have chest pain or increased joint pain, stop. The experts all emphasize: 'Don't overdo it.'

Box 8   *Walking tips*

- If your knees and hips have been severely affected by RA, walking may not be for you. Consider swimming or cycling.
- Warm up for walking by doing range-of-motion exercises for knees and hips.
- Soak your feet in warm water and do range-of-motion foot exercises.
- Wear supportive walking shoes or athletic sneakers with good shock-absorbers.
- Walk on the flat where possible (e.g. beside a river); avoid hills.
- In bad weather walk under cover; those days chopping malls provide miles of covered walking track.
- Swing the arms for balance while walking.
- If your feet feel warm after walking soak them in cool water for ten minutes.

Box 9   *Cycling tips*

- Adjust the seat height of your saddle so that your legs are fully straightened when pedalling.
- Set the handlebars so that they are not too low or far away from the saddle. A prone position puts strain on the lower back, shoulders, elbows and wrists.
- Adjust the pedal tension to the lowest level to limit strain on the knees.
- If the weather is bad try an indoor exercise bike.
- If your knees get painful try an indoor bike with arm motion attachments.
- Cool down with light pedalling as a substitute for range-of-motion exercises.

Turning up the heat

Applying heat may help inflamed joints, and also, conversely, so may applying cold. We've all experienced the comfort of a hot bath or a hot-water bottle when we have aches and pains. There is a sound

---

Box 10 *Swimming tips*

- If possible do a training session under the guidance of a trained physiotherapist.
- Breathe regularly from your diaphragm during exercise.
- Check the temperature of the pool before swimming. Temperatures between 28 and 30°C (82 and 86°F) are best for aerobic exercise. Higher than this increases vasodilatation and may make you feel light-headed. Temperatures up to 33 or 37°C (92 or 98°F) are suitable for range-of-motion and stretching exercise but not for serious swimming.
- Don't go swimming with a temperature, an open wound or if you have a history of uncontrolled seizures, or have either high or low blood pressure.

---

physiological basis for this because local heat causes the blood vessels to expand (*vasodilatation*), increasing the blood-flow to the area and generally speeding up the metabolism. Heat reduces pain, soothes and relaxes mind and body. Although there is no evidence that it has any effect on the progression of RA it does not appear to raise the temperature within inflamed joints.

Heat is especially useful as a prelude to exercise because joints perform better when warmed up. There are a number of different devices for delivering heat, most related to the domestic bath and hot-water bottle. There are whirlpool baths, heat lamps, hot packs and electric heating pads. Heat application can be used in conjunction with gentle range-of-motion exercises as part of your exercise warm-up. (If in the bath do be careful not to cause a flood.) What you use depends on patient preference and what the physiotherapist has available. The best device is one you are happy to use at home. As with exercise, it is important not to overdo heat. Some people have the mistaken idea that hotter is better. It's not. If the skin begins to blotch – as when you have had legs too close to a hot fire – the heat is too great and, no matter how relaxing it is, you should never fall asleep while using heat treatment.

The use of cold is favoured by some physiotherapists. Although it does not have the relaxing, psychological benefits associated with heat, in the case of seriously inflamed swollen joints the benefit of a cold application may be greater than that of heat.

7
Managing pain

Having RA means waking up to pain. Lisa, who has had RA for eight years, tells how it started for her:

> I would wake up in the morning and my feet would really hurt. It would hurt just to walk across the floor. And then I started noticing other symptoms – my hands started to hurt and I couldn't snap my fingers. I would get pain off and on in different joints in my body all day.

The knock-on effect of pain is reduced mobility, wasted muscles, shrinking horizons and a severely curtailed life-style. The medical team naturally focuses upon halting the progress of the disease, knowing that RA can lead to permanently damaged joints, but from the point of view of the patient the first thing to deal with is the pain.

Pain is a complicated thing: a series of messages that travel from one place – usually the site of some injury – through various pathways, using a variety of different bio-chemical processes, to the brain where the pain becomes an experience: 'Ouch!' Reducing or removing pain may therefore be achieved at a number of different points along the chain: from the site of the injury (healing invariably leads to the cessation of pain), to the brain itself: when you are unconscious you feel nothing, including pain. In RA pain is reduced if inflammation is reduced. Further up the line, drugs can interrupt the message travelling to the brain to tell it, 'This hurts'; finally, the brain itself can be taught to reinterpret the message that something is painful and, if not to remove the pain, to lessen its impact and prevent it cowing you into submission. This is what you learn in a pain clinic.

Pain-killers are not sinful

Let us start with taking drugs to reduce pain. Some people are happy to pop a pill every time they have played a strenuous game of tennis or feel the first twinge of toothache or a headache. These people, if they develop RA, will already know which over-the-counter (OTC), easily available pain-killers work for them and which don't. In some ways they are at an advantage in dealing with RA because this is an illness characterized by enduring pain – pain that prevents you doing things and seriously limits your life, but pain that responds quite quickly to those familiar remedies, although they usually have to be taken in much larger quantities than for a headache.

But some are very puritanical about pain-killers; 'Oh, I never take aspirin,' they say, as though swallowing the little white pill was like mainlining on heroin or smoking opium. Stoical attitudes to enduring discomfort and suffering in silence can be deep rooted and are as much cultural as temperamental. The British have a reputation for being long-suffering. In the labour ward British mothers look askance at those from different climes where if it hurts you yell. At funerals they wipe away a furtive tear where other nationalities beat their breasts, tear their hair and let their grief rip.

If you were brought up to think that drugs are bad it's going to be tough to live with an illness that puts you in pain. The very word 'drug' has inevitably become tarnished by bad, harmful drugs. Try telling yourself this: one great difference between our age and the past is that increased understanding has made us better able to prevent, control and cure illness. Without drugs this would not have been possible. Not only drugs, of course – good sanitation and improved nutrition have played their part; but if you arrive at RA with the attitude that drugs are sinful you might as well go back to the dark ages and suffer.

Let us return to the message of pain. In many cases it is extremely important that the message be received. If you touch the hot iron the pain tells your brain; 'That hurts. It's bad for you. Take your finger away.' But what message are your joints sending out when you can hardly put your foot on the floor first thing in the morning? 'Something's wrong; do nothing until it's put right'? In RA the messages have all got muddled up; the inflammatory process is the problem, not the solution. The pain has no meaningful message to give you. So it makes sense to do all you can to stop the pain. Drugs are not the only answer to pain, even in RA. In Chapter 6 we looked at what could be done with exercise and heat. We will also look at psychological techniques that can play a part. But drugs to reduce pain and, in addition, inflammation, are the front-line troops in the battle against RA. They're cheap, they act fast and although they do not appear to modify the progression of the disease they make life bearable while those that do – the DMARDs (see Chapter 8) – take time to clock in.

Aspirin and non-steroidal anti-inflammatory drugs (NSAIDs)

The acronym NSAIDs – pronounced 'en-sayeds' – is used so freely in talking about dear old aspirin and its brothers, used to treat such a wide range of conditions, that it is easy to overlook two important things about them embodied in their name. Yes, they kill pain, but they also reduce inflammation and they do it without belonging to the *cortisone* family of drugs – no, not 'Corleone', though the similarity may make it easier to remember: the *corticosteroids*. Corticosteroids are also powerfully anti-inflammatory, but they pack a bigger pay-load of side effects than NSAIDs (see Chapter 8).

NSAIDs work by interrupting the messages sent from the site of the pain to the brain. The cytokines – the chemical messengers that become so overexcited in RA – produce substances that cause inflammation, called *prostaglandins*. Aspirin and the NSAIDs work by interrupting these processes. That's why you will sometimes hear them called 'prostaglandin-inhibitors'. When production of prostaglandins is reduced so is pain, swelling and stiffness. Doctors prescribe NSAIDs as first-line treatment for RA because they are fast-acting. As anyone who is a fan knows, aspirin offers some pain relief within half an hour. Inflammation and swelling take a little longer, but they start to go down within a matter of a week or so.

However, although they are good at controlling the primary symptoms of RA, NSAIDs do nothing to slow the process of the disease. Because of this doctors often prescribe one of the disease-modifying drugs – DMARDs, second-line treatments – at the same time. These take longer to have an effect but are more beneficial in the long run.

Just as experienced users learn that one pain-killer works better for them than another, so finding the most effective NSAID in RA may also require trial and error. Even NSAIDs (unrelated to the tricky cortisone family) cause some side effects. The most common is indigestion, a result of the fact that the drug irritates the lining of the stomach, which can ultimately lead to ulcers. Recent additions to the NSAID family, called COX-2 inhibitors, seem to have a better side effect profile than older NSAIDs, especially when it comes to stomach irritation (see Box 11 on p. 61). Alternatively, additional medication that reduces acid production in the stomach may be prescribed. If you would like to know more detail of these first-line treatments read on. You may safely take them for granted because most of them have been around some time and their side effects are well known.

Aspirin *(acetylsalicylic acid)*

This drug has been around for more than 100 years, but just because it's old doesn't mean it's not as good as more recent drug discoveries. In fact the list of benefits quoted for aspirin gets longer year by year. It is said to protect against heart disease and even some forms of cancer. In addition it is cheap because it's been around for so long there is no licence premium to pay to the drug company that developed it.

The effects of aspirin are dose-related. Low doses (50 milligrams – mg) a day protect against heart disease; two to three standard pills (600–900 mg) bring down a fever and relieve headache or toothache for up to six hours. But to be effective as an anti-inflammatory in RA aspirin needs to be taken in really high doses – anything from 10 to 20 standard tablets (3 to 6 *grams*) a day. The average dose is usually 4.5 grams (15 tablets) taken every six hours throughout the day with food. The dose is built up gradually because at higher doses this level of aspirin is quite toxic and, quite apart from stomach irritation, some people begin to have ringing in their ears (tinnitus) or slight deafness.

Aspirin may also come wearing fancy-dress

The fancy forms of aspirin are designed to make it act faster or cause fewer side effects. It comes soluble (less irritation than from a hard pill burning itself into the stomach wall wherever it lands). Their tendency to cause stomach irritation is why aspirin and NSAIDs should always be taken with food, never on an empty stomach. Aspirin also comes 'buffered', combined with an ingredient that partially neutralizes stomach acids, and 'film-coated', which makes it easier to swallow; this is not to be confused with *enteric-coated* aspirin which wears a stomach-acid-proof vest that carries it through the stomach and into the small intestine before it dissolves, in order to reduce the risk of both indigestion, irritation and ulcers in the stomach. Inevitably the coating interferes with the rate at which the pay-load is absorbed. Finally, aspirin may come in a coat that makes it dissolve little by little – a time-release capsule. It reduces some, but not all, of the side effects of the drug and also cuts down the number of times it must be taken each day. All these fancy formulations add to the cost of the medicine.

The side effects of aspirin

Some people have to avoid aspirin even as a headache pill, so before putting an RA patient on high-dose aspirin the good doctor checks for any contraindications – evidence in the patient's history that suggests that he or she may react badly to the drug. Apart from indigestion, gut irritation or evidence of ulcers, a history of asthma, nasal polyps, kidney or liver problems are all warning signs. Some people are actually allergic to aspirin. A number of other drugs can interact with aspirin, especially those taken for various forms of heart or circulatory disease that thin the blood. This is because in addition to inhibiting the production of prostaglandins, aspirin reduces the number of *platelets* in the bloodstream (platelets are part of the blood-clotting mechanism, so this is the reason aspirin increases bleeding in the gut and a tendency to bruise). This is actually beneficial in heart disease but too much of a good thing if you are already taking medication specifically to reduce blood-clotting. The doctor will also check for whether the patient smokes or drinks alcohol because these also irritate the stomach.

NSAIDs

NSAIDs cause fewer gastric problems than aspirin and have a similarly beneficial effect on the primary symptoms of RA. The oldest – indomethacin – has been around for 40 years and consequently costs less than new, on-licence versions of the drug. Some, such as ibuprofen, can also be bought OTC at a chemist, like aspirin. It goes without saying that all drugs taken to treat RA must be taken in consultation with a doctor even if they are available off-prescription.

There is little difference in how well the numerous NSAIDs reduce inflammation. They cause similar side effects to aspirin – gut irritation, possible ulcers and gastric bleeding – and in order to reduce these, drug firms have produced similar fancy-dress versions: soluble, enteric-coated, slow-release and buffered with something that counteracts their effect on the stomach lining. But although there is little difference in their overall effectiveness, there is considerable difference in how individual patients respond to particular drugs. About two-thirds of patients respond to any NSAID, but it may take considerable trial and error to find an effective drug for patients in the remaining third. NSAIDs are based on a number of different chemicals, and if no result is achieved with one sort after three weeks, one with a different chemical make-up will be tried until one that works is found.

For information on drug names, see Box 12 on p. 63.

Box 11   *COX inhibitors*

NSAIDs do not loom as large as the DMARDs in the great scheme of RA treatment. But NSAIDs are widely prescribed for a whole range of medical problems and it is estimated that as many as 30 million people worldwide take NSAIDs every day to control their pain and inflammation. They work by blocking an enzyme known as *cyclo-oxygenase* (COX). This enzyme contributes to the production of beneficial prostaglandins which release platelets that protect the gut, kidneys and blood. But just over 12 years ago scientists discovered that inflamed tissues contained increased amounts of the COX enzyme and that the extra COX was different from that found in tissue that was not inflamed. We now had COX-1 and COX-2. COX-2 is produced in response to stimulation by those overexcited cytokines. In crude terms COX-1, which acts to protect the gastric lining, was the good guy and COX-2, produced only in inflamed tissue, was the bad guy. The race was on to inhibit COX-2 while leaving COX-1 to carry on protecting. Three drugs that inhibit COX-2 selectively are now available and others are in developments. There is still some overlap effect on COX-1, but in clinical trials of people with arthritis these improved NSAIDs were shown to control pain and inflammation without nasty side effects in the stomach.

Rowland's story

Rowland had been on RA medication for some months when he noticed strange marks on the palms of his hands. He was a self-employed carpenter and had tried to keep working as best he could in spite of his illness. He was doing his exercises and the NSAID the doctor had prescribed had reduced the pain and swelling, but he still had a lot of problems managing his tools. He showed his hands to the doctor. 'It looks like a bruise,' he said. The doctor examined his body and found similar bruises on the pressure points on the soles of his feet and at various parts of his arms and legs where he must have knocked himself. He asked Rowland to bring in a sample of his stool and discovered dark, tarry stuff in it caused by excessive bleeding from the gut. Even before he saw the stool, the doctor realized that Rowland was reacting to the high-dose NSAID prescribed to reduce pain and inflammation. He stopped the drug and started Roland on a new COX-2 inhibitor, celecoxib. Roland's bruising cleared up but he had learned to be very careful not to knock or put excessive pressure on his skin.

Pain management programmes

Modern pain-killing drugs are amazing. They are so good that it is tempting to forget that there are times when they don't work. In 90 per cent of cases of RA the drugs we have described in this chapter will, if not eliminate pain, at least bring it under control. But it would be dishonest to tell you that this is guaranteed.

Because the management of pain with drugs has such a successful history it is easy to think that they are the only way of dealing with chronic or persistent pain. And a rheumatologist faced with an RA patient who is still seriously handicapped by pain when all the various NSAIDs and COX-2 drugs have been tried will probably suggest more powerful pills or a course of injections to try and control the pain.

However, this is not the only option.

The problem of chronic and persistent pain is not unique to RA. It is occurs in many non-fatal medical conditions. In RA the origin of pain is known and can be addressed. But in some situations pain may have no clear explanation and may continue for months – or even for life. Sometimes multiple investigations will have found no cause; nevertheless, the effects of chronic pain can be devastating.

In response to the need for something other than or in addition to drugs to treat intractable pain a network of specialist pain clinics has started to appear. These pain clinics are usually part of a hospital

Box 12 *On drug names*

Drug names belong to no spoken language and are almost impossible to pronounce and remember. They are assembled piecemeal by the people who develop the drugs and are intended to provide clues as to what's in them or how they work. But they only do this for experienced pharmacists. Just to complicate matters, each drug has at least two names: its generic name – this is the name that describes its active ingredients – and its trade name. Trade names are meant to be catchy and easier to pronounce than chemical names, but they often aren't. Trade names vary from country to country. This makes it very difficult for the lay person to recognize what it is he is taking. There is an unspoken belief among doctors that patients don't really need to know more about their drugs than is included in the Patient Information Leaflet enclosed in the pack – with the apt acronym PIL. They think it will make you worry. But if you know the names of your drug and can get on to the internet you can find out a fantastic amount, both good and bad, about your medication. Here are some of the names of aspirins and NSAIDs commonly prescribed as first-line treatment for RA, just in case you want to do this. In each group the name of the generic compound is followed by various trade names. This is by no means an exhaustive list of aspirin and NSAID drugs.

Aspirin	acetylsalicylic acid (aspirin, Aspro Clear, Bufferin, Ecotrin, Encaprin)
NSAID	indomethacin (Orudis, Orudis KT, Actron, Oruvail)
	ibuprofen (Motrin, Advil, Advin, Medipren, Midol, Motrin)
	naproxen (Naprosyn)
	diclofenac (Voltaren, Voltaren XL, Cataflam)
	oxaprozin (Daypro)
	fenbufen (Fenoprofen, Naflon)
	ketoprofen
COX-2 inhibitors	meloxicam (Mobic)
	celecoxib (Celebrex)

out-patient department and they vary in the treatment they offer. They usually work with patients in groups and employ a team of doctors, psychologists, nurses, physiotherapists, psychotherapists and occupational therapists who approach the pain from all directions to overcome the disability it causes, if not the pain itself. For example, training in how you move and hold yourself can dramatically reduce pain; learning how to pick things up and otherwise handle objects can reduce pain. This is the domain of the physiotherapist or occupational therapist. (More of them in Chapter 12.)

The psychotherapists work by exploiting the final link in the pain message, where it is received in the brain. It is known that people experience pain differently depending on temperament and on the situation they are in. Amazing examples of soldiers who kept going in spite of broken limbs because it was their only chance of escape illustrate this. Psychologists have developed techniques known broadly as *cognitive behaviour therapy* which teach you how to change the way you register pain and react to it by changing the way you think. Instead of 'Ain't it awful; I can't bear it,' you learn: 'That's pain; so what? I'm not going to let it get in the way of what I want to do.'

It is not possible to say definitively how many people may be helped by going through a pain management programme. By definition they are only there because their pain is intractable and resistant to most pain-killers. Also, the goal is not to cure the pain so much as to make the patient able to put it on one side and get on with their life. Most people benefit to some degree from the training. A patient who had taken part in the hundredth pain management programme at the Pain Management Unit attached to the Royal National Hospital for Rheumatic Diseases in Bath said this: '*I can't* has become *I certainly can!*'

You can find out more about pain clinics from the British Pain Society among others; contact details are listed in Useful addresses, at the end of the book.

8

Drugs that change the course of the disease

Just to remind you: the acronym DMARDs stands for disease-modifying anti-rheumatic drugs, and the key word in that name is 'modifying'. Exercise will maintain the maximum possible function in RA-affected joints; aspirin or NSAIDs will reduce the pain and inflammation, modifying the way you think and feel about things and the way you organize your life (see Chapters 10 and 11), and will minimize the way RA affects the rest of your life. But none of these alters the course of the disease. The damage and eventual erosion of joints continues.

But the group called DMARDs go one better: they not only treat symptoms, they interrupt the progress of RA. Some of these drugs have been around treating other conditions for some time and were serendipitously discovered to be beneficial in RA. Gold (strictly speaking, gold salts) was introduced in the 1920s to treat tuberculosis; chloroquine is prescribed to protect against malaria; penicillamine is a break-down product of one of the earliest antibiotics, penicillin; and methotrexate, which damps down the immune system (it is *immunosuppressant*), is used to treat some cancers. Azathioprine has a similar effect on the immune system and is used after a transplant operation to prevent the body rejecting the transplant. In fact, of the older drugs only sulfasalazine – an anti-inflammatory which contains salicylic acids, like aspirin, and an antibacterial compound – was specifically designed to treat arthritis. First used in the 1940s, it has come into increasing prominence in the last 20 years. Studies show that, overall, it is marginally more effective compared with most of the others. Cyclosporine, another drug first used to prevent transplant rejections, came into use in the 1970s, and leflunomide, actually designed for RA, was only introduced in 1999. These drugs may be used one at a time, in succession or, if that is not effective, in combination.

Beth's mother's story
Beth lived in fear of RA for years before she was diagnosed at 18, because her youth had been overshadowed by her mother's severe RA.

'When it's in the family it is like a black cloud on the horizon; you don't know if the cloud-burst will move over or come down on top of you. My teenage daughter now feels the same way. I had seen what injecting gold had done to my mother, and massive doses of steroids. That's all they had in those days. She was housebound for nearly four years. I remember going down to the library and bringing back about eight novels a day for her to read. I had to go out and buy my own school uniform. It gave me a very sceptical attitude to RA drugs.'

Powerful, effective, but dangerous to know

Each DMARD is chemically distinct. Not all of them are directly anti-inflammatory; some work by suppressing the immune system and it is possible that these drugs interfere with disease by reducing the overexcited white cells that are produced in such great numbers

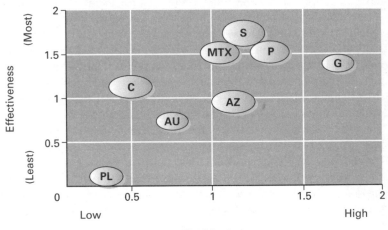

Figure 5 The effectiveness of DMARDs
Key: PL = placebo; AU = oral gold; AZ = azathioprine;
C = chloroquine and hydroxychloroquine; MTX = methotrexate;
S = sulfasalazine; P = penicillamine; G = injected gold

Source Adapted from D. T. Felson *et al.*, 'The comparative efficacy and toxicity of second-line drugs in rheumatoid arthritis: results of two meta-analyses', *Arthritis and Rheumatism*, 33 (10), pp. 1449–61, 1990.

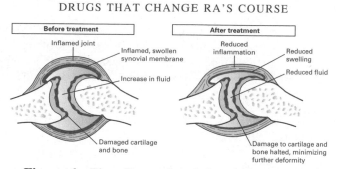

Figure 6   The effects of anti-rheumatic medicines

that they start to damage the lining of the joints. To be frank, no one is quite sure why they work in RA, but they do. In most cases they achieve at least a slowing down of damage inflicted by inflammation on the joints. In some cases they achieve complete remission. Figure 5 shows the effectiveness of DMARDs compared with their toxicity, and Figure 6 compares a joint before and after treatment with DMARDs.

These drugs are slow-acting (they are sometimes known as Slow-Acting Anti-Rheumatic drugs – SAARDs) but all are powerful and effective at the right dose even if their method of action is mysterious. If you are diagnosed with RA it is vital you know something about them because 50 per cent of rheumatology departments in the UK now start patients on DMARDs as soon as the diagnosis is confirmed. In addition, they can have quite severe side effects, which means that the drug you start on may have to be changed until you find one that suits you. **All DMARDs are contraindicated in pregnancy and during breast-feeding.**

Gold salts (aurothiomalate)

Gold can be administered by injection into a muscle or taken as a pill by mouth. It is marginally more effective as an injection, and patients can be taught how to give themselves the injections, as diabetics do. However, there are more side effects when gold is taken this way. The patient is started on a low dose and it is increased gradually over several weeks until the effective dose is achieved, probably after about five or six weeks. (The same goes for gold taken in tablet form.) Three-quarters of patients experience a reduction in swelling and rheumatoid nodules, but half also have some side effects. These include rashes, reaction to sunlight, diarrhoea, and possible damage to the kidneys and (rarely) to the important clotting platelets in the blood. The blood and urine of anyone taking gold is monitored constantly for signs of these side effects, and if any untreatable symptoms appear the drug is stopped.

Penicillamine

This has been in use for RA since the 1960s and is taken by mouth, daily, in gradually increasing doses. Again, it takes some weeks to build up to an effective dose and it can be as much as nine months before it has any effect on the progress of RA. Some groups of people react badly to the drug. This reaction is no more common among those who are allergic to the antibiotic penicillin, even though the two drugs are related. Nowadays there are safer DMARDs available so penicillamine is rarely prescribed, and then only under very close supervision.

Chloroquine and hydroxychloroquine

These pills are swallowed daily and take between six weeks and six months to take effect. The active ingredient in them is quinine, known for centuries to have healing properties and best known as a protection against malaria. (There is quinine in tonic water, which is said to explain the popularity of gin and tonic among expatriates living in India, Africa and the Far East.) Quinine drugs have been used to treat RA patients since the 1950s. Their effectiveness is roughly on a par with injected gold salts, but they have a better side effect profile. Most side effects – skin rashes, nausea and diarrhoea – disappear if the dose is reduced. The only serious risk with long-term use is that of damage to the eyes (*retinopathy*), but this is rare with the doses of hydroxy-chloroquine that are usually prescribed for RA. Just occasionally when you first take the drugs you may have slightly blurred vision. This is not a sign that you are going blind. It usually clears within a week. However, the risk is sufficient to require that you have an eye-test before taking quinine drugs so that a base-line can be established against which your eyes may be checked during treatment. Hydroxy-chloroquine may be combined successfully with other DMARDs.

Sulfasalazine

This drug was developed in the 1930s for RA at a time when the disease was considered to be caused by an infection. (It contains an early antibiotic – sulfa – as well as the anti-inflammatory salicylate.)

It fell into disfavour when the new, miraculous anti-inflammatory properties of the corticosteroids were discovered, but made a comeback when the down-side of the risky cortisone family was revealed. (In the USA it was not licensed for the treatment of RA until 1996.) In terms of effectiveness it rates with, or slightly above, methotrexate, with a similar level of side effects. Sulfasalazine is taken twice a day in enteric-coated tablets so that it will pass through the stomach without causing irritation and be absorbed in the bowel. As with other DMARDs the dose is increased gradually until the effective level is found. It starts to take effect in two to six months. In spite of the enteric coating some 20 per cent of those taking the drug suffer some form of stomach upset, although this can be minimized by taking the pills with food and taking additional drugs to counteract this effect. Very occasionally people are allergic to the sulfa in the drug, but this clears up once the medication is discontinued. It also reduces the sperm count. Again this is temporary and returns to normal when treatment is discontinued.

The last four drugs in this pharmacy act by suppressing the immune system.

Methotrexate

This is regarded by many doctors as one of the most effective DMARDs available in the relatively low doses prescribed for RA. It has been used in very high doses to treat cancer since the 1940s but since the 1980s has zoomed to the top of the charts for RA. Its popularity is based on its effectiveness – only exceeded by sulfasalazine: it acts rapidly for a DMARD, with results sometimes in two weeks and invariably by eight, is taken weekly and increased in stages until the therapeutic dose is achieved, and it has fewer side effects than injected gold, penicillamine, sulfasalazine and azathioprine. It still has side effects: nausea is the most common; vomiting, rash, diarrhoea and headache are occasionally reported. But its effect on the immune system, on the bone-marrow and the liver means that patients require very close monitoring when they are on it. Under these circumstances patients have remained on the drug for three to five years.

Azathioprine

This drug is also used to treat cancer and to avoid the body rejecting a transplanted organ. It becomes effective between six weeks and six months, but like methotrexate its effect on the immune system can be severe, leaving the patient vulnerable to infection. Most doctors only prescribe it if other DMARDs have failed, or in combination with other drugs.

Cyclosporine

This group of strongly immunosuppressive medicines was discovered in the 1970s. It was developed to suppress transplant rejections but is now prescribed as a DMARD for severe, active RA. It is usually taken twice a day and can be effective after four to eight weeks. Doctors tend to prescribe it, like azathioprine, when methotrexate has not been satisfactory or in combination with other drugs. It has an effect on kidney function in almost half those who take it – quite seriously in some. It also causes high blood pressure, as well as a number of minor side effects. It is not a DMARD of first choice. Nevertheless, some of those who can tolerate it have been on it for as long as five years.

Leflunomide

This DMARD only came on to the market five years ago. It is called an *immunomodulator* because it has a selective effect on parts of the immune system that promote inflammation. Comparative studies indicate that, over a year, its effect on the primary arthritic symptoms is roughly the same as methotrexate or sulfasalazine, although it works for slightly fewer patients (51 per cent against 65 per cent for methotrexate). Those who took it reported that their physical functioning was marginally better than with the established drugs. Its side effects are similar to those of the other drugs with the additional risk of liver damage, so that anyone taking it is very closely monitored. It is too soon to know whether it will be tolerated with prolonged use. Being a new drug it is a great deal more expensive than older DMARDs.

Side-effects of DMARDs

Nausea is the miserable trademark of taking DMARDs for most patients. 'You almost get used to it,' said Beth.

A bit like morning sickness. I remember taking the children to school, having taken my pills at breakfast. It was always – *oh God, will I manage to get home without throwing up?* I was considered a failure on methotrexate. Nowadays I take hydroxychloroquine and sulfasalazine. I still feel sick sometimes – perhaps not as often.

Lisa's story
Lisa, who now runs self-help classes for the US Arthritis Foundation, also had an initially bad experience with DMARDs.

'I was started on a series of drugs which are supposed to halt the disease from progressing any further, to prevent you from getting twisted joints and disfigured hands. I was started on methotrexate and oral gold, but I ended up having a bad photosensitive reaction to the gold (I was out in the sun and everything I looked at turned silver and I got bad hives and ended up having to go to the ER) . . . Since I've been diagnosed, my regimen has changed a couple different times for different reasons. After I had the reaction to the gold, I went on sulfasalazine and Plaquenil [hydroxychloroquine]. I was on those for a while and then I had a reaction to the sulfasalazine. Then I went on a drug called Enbrel, which is one of a newer class of drugs called biologic agents [see Chapter 9]. For the past 8–10 months I have been giving myself injections of Enbrel twice a week and that was like a wonder drug – I felt really good on it. But now that my husband and I are trying to get pregnant, I'm only on prednisone [a corticosteroid – see below], because Enbrel is contraindicated for pregnancy.'

How long will you have to take DMARDs?

The slowness of DMARDs is a major source of frustration to both doctor and patient, especially as you may have to change from one to another if you develop one of the severe side effects. If you finally find one that works and the disease slows down, stops even, should you keep taking it, or risk stopping and having a flare-up and then having to go through the whole lengthy process again?

Medical opinion has long been divided on the wisdom of taking anything as powerful and disruptive to the body's functioning as a DMARD indefinitely. But recently some studies have been published showing that those who come off DMARDs are twice as likely to have a flare-up within a year than those who continue treatment. The verdict appears to be 'Keep on taking the tablets.'

Corticosteroids in RA

Human steroids are natural hormones produced mostly by the adrenal glands, but also by the testicles and ovaries. They help control *metabolism* – that's how the body generates energy and disposes of waste – the development of sexual characteristics, immune function, the balance of fluids in the body and its tolerance of stress. There are many steroids with different functions: the sex hormones – testosterone, oestrogen and progesterone – adrenal cortical hormones, bile acids, sterols, anabolic agents and oral contraceptives are all steroids. Pay attention now: corticosteroids are not the same as anabolic steroids, the ones taken by weightlifters to build muscle. The role of corticosteroids is protective: they maintain the fluid balance in the body and help it cope with stress; along the way they reduce inflammation.

Corticosteroid drugs are chemical versions of the hormones produced naturally in the body. When cortisone was discovered in the 1940s it demonstrated such dramatic reductions in inflammation that it was hailed as a wonder drug – a 'cure' for RA – and earned its discoverers, Philip Hench and Edward Kendall, a Nobel Prize.

But in the wake of the rave reviews for the miracle cure came serious side effects – especially because the drugs were being used in high doses at this time: weight-gain, raised blood pressure, easy bruising and slow healing, cataracts, muscular weakness, raised blood-sugar causing problems with diabetes, less resistance to infection because the immune system was being damped down and, over long-term use, thinning of the bones – osteoporosis. Suddenly corticosteroids were no longer flavour of the month. Beth's mother received massive injections of cortisone during the 1950s. She now takes medication for the osteoporosis it caused in addition to all her drugs for RA.

Modern uses of corticosteroids

Over time the pros and cons of corticosteroids have become better understood, their use, delivery and dosage refined. These days they once again have a role to play in RA but doctors follow strict guidelines. They are usually used short-term, in emergencies – for example if inflammation of the blood vessels – vasculitis – is affecting nerves or important organs. If they are taken by mouth the lowest dose is taken for the shortest possible period to produce a reduction in inflammation. They can also be used to reduce inflammation while waiting for slow-acting DMARDs to cut in. This is called bridge therapy, for obvious reasons. They are (see Lisa's story on p. 71) relatively safe to use during pregnancy. When corticosteroids have been prescribed the dose must be reduced gradually, not stopped abruptly, and under medical supervision. When they are phased out the short-term side effects – bloating, the dreaded nausea and mood changes – stop too. (See Box 13 for a list of some corticosteroid drugs.)

One of the most successful uses of corticosteroids is as an anti-inflammatory injection, directly into an affected joint. Localized use of the drug in this way does not carry the same side effects as taking it by mouth. Great care has to be taken when injecting drugs into a joint; sterile conditions must be observed to avoid the risk of introducing infection and it requires considerable skill to position the needle so that its load is delivered into the joint without injuring surrounding tendons or other structures. For this reason only experienced doctors, usually those working in a rheumatology department, attempt it.

If you receive an intra-articular injection (into the joint) you will probably be offered an anaesthetic to numb the skin beforehand. Immediately afterwards an ice-pack on the joint will speed the action of the drug. You will probably be advised to rest the joint for at least 48 hours and avoid putting any strain on it for a week or two. Corticosteroid injections can safely be repeated after about four months.

Box 13   *Names of some corticosteroid drugs*

Hydrocortisone, cortisone, prednisone, prednisolone, methylprednisolone, triamcinolone, betamethazone, dexamethazone and rimexolone.

9

Bio-medicines that fine-tune
the immune response

In the last chapter we explained that many of the drugs that affect the progress of RA – the DMARDs – were originally used to treat something else and were discovered to work in RA by accident. Drug research is a bit like that. Bio-medicines, or *biologics* as they are also known, are not like that. They are a product of scientists' increasingly sophisticated understanding of the inflammatory process. As yet, they don't know what sparks it off in RA – that will come – but they know a great deal about the small steps in the progression that leads from initial inflammatory response inside the joint to the mass production – *proliferation* – of cytokines and cells of the immune system, and eventually to the destruction of cartilage and bone in affected joints.

The name the doctors give to this step-by-step process is 'cascade'. It conjures up a useful image: if you imagine water pouring over an edge into a pool below, and, once the pool below is filled, overflowing into another pool below that, and so on and so on, you have an idea of how one thing leads to another in the human body. You can also imagine how many different targets such a system offers for breaking the chain and interrupting the process. Drug developers like the word 'target', too. You can (figuratively) turn off the water at the source; mop it up; divert it; cover the pools so it can't get in, or raise the sides of the pools so it can't get out. Similar opportunities are being exploited by drug developers trying to stop the progress of RA.

Biological treatments for RA have only become available in the past ten years, yet already it is clear that, short of prevention and the Holy Grail of a vaccine against the disease, these are the drugs that really deliver results – not yet cure, but they certainly control RA. Because of this it's worth taking a little effort to understand how they work. Many more are in development and almost certainly by the time this book appears more will have come on to the market.

The blunderbuss versus the rapier

Old drugs tended to hit the body with a blunt instrument: they knocked out unhealthy and healthy tissue alike, or they blocked a whole system, losing good functions as well as bad. New biological drugs are targeted more precisely. In Chapter 7 we described the new COX-2 inhibitors which are able to reduce inflammatory prostaglandins while leaving beneficial ones available to maintain the blood's clotting mechanism; in the same way, bio-medicines aim to remove the harmful activities of the parts of the immune system that go haywire in RA while not depriving the body of their protective action. These new targeted drugs are like a rapier in contrast to the old blunderbuss drugs.

Bio-medicines work by imitating natural processes and natural materials. They are man-made, like chemical drugs, but from small pieces of living tissue called *proteins*. Being made of protein makes them difficult to deliver via the mouth because they would be broken down by the acids in the stomach, which digests protein, so they are usually injected straight into the bloodstream.

Interrupting the message or reprogramming the messengers

To understand how bio-medicines work it is necessary to return to that cascade of inflammatory and destructive events that mark the progress of RA. In Chapter 2 we explained how in the healthy immune system inflammatory T and B lymphocytes, neutrophils and macrophages are produced to fight infection or repair damage. In RA an unknown trigger stimulates these immune cells to be mass produced and then to start clumping together. The instruction to do this is communicated by chemical messengers called cytokines, and in RA, lacking an external invader, the immune cells start attacking the cartilage and bone in the joint.

Different cytokines deliver different messages. Two that are known to deliver the inflammation message are tumour necrosis factor (TNF) and interleukin-1 (IL-1). But other cytokines carry messages to damp the process down. In addition it must be remembered that TNF and IL-1 play a beneficial role in fighting genuine outsiders so we don't want to kill them off completely. The goal is to correct the balance between the pro- and anti-inflammatory cytokines by decreasing the one or increasing the other. This gives the bio-engineers a choice of targets.

They can prevent the inflammatory message being delivered by blocking the place where the cytokines post the message to the immune cells. The docking-site is known as a receptor, and a drug that can plug this receptor is called a *receptor antagonist*. A medical antagonist is not unlike a human one: it is against you, or in this case against IL-1 getting to home base. An example of this sort of bio-medicine is a very recent biologic agent called anakinra (Kineret) – see p. 80 – which plugs up the docking-site (receptor) for IL-1. Receptor antagonists for TNF are also being studied.

Another approach is to intercept the messages carried by the inflammation cytokines and mop them up while they are in transit. The body produces free-ranging proteins called soluble receptors which can attach themselves to inflammation messages and prevent them reaching port. It produces increased numbers of these in an attempt to control inflammation by mopping up these messages. A successful new bio-drug called etanercept (Enbrel) – see Lisa's story in Chapter 8 – mimics the action of these soluble receptors and captures TNF before it can dock with immune cells and deliver its instructions.

Other biologics tackle the source of the inflammatory messages by neutralizing inflammatory cytokines with man-made antibodies specially designed to disable them. These antibodies are known as *monoclonal antibodies* (MoAbs). There are MoAbs targeted on TNF – infliximab (Remicade) and adalimumab (Humira) – rare examples of drug names that actually tell you something about what's in them. MoAbs can be engineered to capture a wide range of targets and are proving a very promising line of drug development.

Receiving biologic therapy

Biologic treatments for RA work fast (etanercept and infliximab both take between two weeks and three months) and have a relatively low side effect profile. The only serious one is that because they act on TNF – part of the immune system – resistance to infection is depressed while someone is taking them. All potential patients are screened for contact with TB before being selected. But biologics are still quite new – etanercept, the oldest, came on to the market only six years ago – and the least expensive costs more than three times as much as the most expensive DMARD (£10,000 for a year's supply against £3,000 for cyclosporine). For all these reasons biologics are usually prescribed only for RA patients who have failed to respond to established medication, or to those with extremely severe symptoms. In some cases a biologic treatment may be used in conjunction with a DMARD like methotrexate. Occasionally the biologic is used as a first-line treatment when a patient is in the early stages of RA but shows signs of having a rapidly progressing form of the disease.

Cost apart, biologic medicines are highly effective. Etanercept not only reduces joint pain, swelling and stiffness, but people who have taken it say they have more energy and improved day-to-day functioning and there is good evidence that it also delays the structural damage caused by RA. Long-term studies suggest the benefit may be continuous.

Do-it-yourself injections . . .

Drugs made from proteins are similar in some ways to food proteins. They cannot be swallowed as pills because the stomach would digest them before they had a chance to become effective. They have to be delivered direct to the bloodstream.

Etanercept is given by *subcutaneous* (under the skin) injection twice weekly. Experts in the rheumatology department teach patients how to do this for themselves, at home. Sticking a needle into yourself can seem daunting to the initiated. (See Box 5, p. 34.) It's one thing to steel yourself to the medical team treating you like a pin-cushion, it's quite another to do the deed yourself. But, like millions of diabetics, you eventually become quite sanguine about it. Ideally someone living with you should also learn to give the injection in case your hands are ever too sore. (See Lisa in Chapter 8.) Like insulin, another biologic treatment, etanercept is damaged by high or very low temperatures and has to be stored at between 2 and 8°C. An insulated cool-bag will be needed if you plan to travel with this sort of medication.

Preparing, administering and looking after biologic medication is quite tricky, and so is using and disposing of hypodermic needles. These days all needles are single-use, throw-away. But you may be sure that the medical team take every care to ensure that you are thoroughly trained before they will let you out of the hospital with their expensive, vulnerable medicine. In the USA the manufacturers of etanercept run a support programme for users called Enliven, with a newsletter and free helpline, also called Enliven. At the moment the service is not available in the UK.

... *or have it done for you*

Like etanercept, infliximab (Remicade) blocks the cytokine TNF, but it does so by means of a specially engineered monoclonal antibody (the 'mab' bit of its name) that latches on to the cytokine and prevents it spreading its inflammation message. Like etanercept, infliximab can produce results within two weeks and is usually effective within three months. Increased susceptibility to infection is its only major side effect, and while they are on the course patients are very closely monitored.

Infliximab is another new, expensive drug and only the same special groups of patients – the unresponsive, the seriously affected or those whose RA is rapidly progressing – are likely to receive it. It also has to be delivered directly into the bloodstream, in this case by a technique called infusion that can only be done in hospital out-patients.

In infusion a lead is introduced into a vein – rather as it is to draw blood during donation or when someone is put on to a saline drip – and the medicine is introduced slowly over a period of about two hours. The second infusion is given a fortnight later and the third after another three weeks, and thereafter at six- to eight-week intervals. At the moment it is usually used in combination with methotrexate and in this regimen is very successful at reducing the signs and symptoms of RA and slowing down joint damage.

Because these drugs are new and very expensive not many RA patients have yet received them. Those who have been lucky are unreservedly enthusiastic about them, in spite of the fact that RA patients, like Beth, sceptical and resigned through two generations of RA suffering, are under no illusions about the down-side of the medication that they are prescribed. They have heard the story of corticosteroids. Wonder-drugs sometimes have feet of clay. Only time truly tells.

Effective treatments, but not available to all

Sharon's story

Sharon (not her real name) was fortunate enough to be selected to take place in clinical trials for the early biologic agents. She decided to write a detailed account of the experience and send it to her local arthritis support organization in the hope that publicizing her personal success story might galvanize rheumatologists around the country to badger those in charge of drug funding to find more money so that these expensive drug treatments could be prescribed for more RA patients. She says:

'My RA started four years ago and did not respond well to any of the conventional treatments. It was deemed an aggressive form. After years of trauma when the drug treatments failed, in September 2002 I started on the infusion treatment and my RA has been in recession since spring 2003. I cannot thank my local arthritis clinic enough and also my local Health Authority for all they have done for me. I believe that while there is no cure for RA, everybody should have at least the chance to take part in the biological treatments. I have talked with people, who have had RA for 20 years or more, who could only walk on two crutches and who are now walking normally and unaided. For that reason, it is necessary to collect more and more signatures to persuade those in charge of the purse-strings that people with RA deserve a better quality of life and to be able to live pain-free lives.'

Sharon describes what is involved in having an infusion.

'The infliximab infusion is prepared on the day of the patient's arrival, with the powder form measured out based on the patient's weight. At first the patient is given a saline solution, then the infusion solution and finally another saline solution to flush the infliximab through. There are rules about how fast the drip can run, and it is constantly monitored to adjust the flow. During the session the patient's blood pressure is continuously measured, and at least one doctor comes to listen to the patient's heart-rate. Patients will also be asked questions and may have their joints examined.'

Christine's story

Christine had to go into battle like a gladiator to get expensive biologic treatment.

'As soon as I knew it [infliximab] had been passed by NICE [the National Institute for Clinical Excellence, which evaluates treatments and care for effectiveness] I approached my rheumatologist to see if I could have the drug. I was told that the hospital couldn't afford it and that there was no funding available. I was determined that I was not going to take no for an answer so I lobbied every MP in the area who would have patients visiting the hospital. My own constituency MP was very helpful and I wrote letters to the Department of Health and the hospital management. I also had a half-hour on our local radio station who also lobbied the hospital. Four days later I got a telephone call telling me I could have the drug.

'I had my first infusion at the end of October and within four days I was 98 per cent pain-free. Because of the joint damage that I have I am still disabled but to be pain-free is a 100 per cent improvement on my quality of life. I have now had my fourth infusion and have been told that I can carry on with the treatment. I'm even more delighted that I am now seeing other people at the hospital who are having infusions.

'So, if you have been turned down for this drug – please do what I did! No one should be in excruciating pain when there is a drug which will alleviate it. You deserve this drug.'

More biologics joining the field

A third biologic agent has been licensed in the USA and more recently in the UK. It's called anakinra (Kineret) and unlike its predecessors it works not against TNF but by blocking another major inflammatory cytokine – interleukin-1 (IL-1). This cytokine has been identified as the dominant player in the destructive processes of RA. Anakinra blocks the docking-sites (receptors) for IL-1 so that it cannot deliver its inflammation message. It is a man-made protein modelled on a naturally occurring protein called interleukin-1-receptor antagonist (IL-1RA).

Anakinra is given once a day by subcutaneous injection by means of a pre-filled syringe: no mixing necessary. The studies done during its development suggest it is effective on a par with its biologic predecessors, with a similar side effect profile: the nuisance of reactions at the site of the injection and the serious one of an increased susceptibility to infection.

It is, of course, also very expensive and to date the regulatory agencies in this country and in Europe are reluctant to recommend it because it does not seem to offer any advance on existing medication.

Other biologic treatments are in development and may have been launched on the market by the time this book appears. At £10,000 a year, and rising, to treat one patient, these treatments have a lot to prove, and they will need to offer major advances over etanercept and infliximab to persuade the cost-conscious drug purchasers in the National Health Service that they provide value for money.

Warning note

Serious though rare side effects are a known disadvantage of many powerful new drugs. Inevitably, as greater numbers use a drug, uncommon side effects start to emerge. The manufacturer of infliximab has recently warned health professionals in the USA that a number of patients worldwide have suffered potentially fatal blood disorders and that there have also been complications affecting the central nervous system. Changes are being made to the prescribing and patient advice for infliximab. Product information in the EU already tells those who prescribe medicines to monitor patients on infliximab for any sign of these problems.

10

Serious manifestations of RA and surgery

It would be dishonest to write about RA without dealing with the serious manifestations of the disease that afflict about 5 per cent of sufferers. In the past more people had to endure this experience of RA. As understanding and treatment progress, the hope is that fewer and fewer people will be badly affected, but it would be unrealistic to hope that such outcomes will become a thing of the past in our lifetime: there are still many people whose disease progressed before the arrival of today's advanced drug treatments, let alone the improved treatments of the future.

Meet the surgeon

If you have RA you will have become familiar with hospitals. Sophisticated diagnostic tests, monitoring, specialist clinics, therapists and the delivery of advanced medication all take place in the rheumatology department of the hospital. If you reach the steeper slopes of RA you will move over to a surgical department. You are usually recommended for surgery on the advice of the rheumatology specialist. Surgeons who specialize in bone or joint operations are known as *orthopaedic* surgeons. (See the glossary for the curious origins of this name.)

There are a number of procedures a surgeon can perform to help someone with advanced RA. There are minor procedures which provide temporary relief or which aim to ward off long-term damage. Others are adopted to correct or replace joints which have already been seriously damaged. The most common reason for surgery is to control intractable (unresponsive to other treatments) pain caused by inflammation or damaged joints. But surgeons can also repair ruptured ligaments or tendons; they may remove synovial tissue from a joint that has not responded to treatment; they may fuse (join together) the bones of a joint (for more on spontaneous fusion, see Box 14 opposite); and finally they may replace the joint completely with a man-made joint. A replacement joint or any artificial body-part is known as a *prosthesis*.

The replacement of painful and damaged joints – caused most commonly by OA – is becoming a more frequent and successful operation and there are now more centres in the UK where it is carried out. But the joints affected and replaced for OA are principally the knee and hip. Orthopaedic surgeons who specialize in the hands or feet – more frequently affected by RA – are a little thinner on the ground. The rheumatologist who refers you is best placed to know where the most experienced specialists can be found. You are perfectly entitled to ask how many operations like the one proposed for you the surgeon has previously carried out. Surgeons carrying out novel procedures, unlike drugs, do not have to go through lengthy clinical trials before they can be licensed for use on patients.

Box 14 *Spontaneous fusion*

The fusion of an RA-affected joint can occur spontaneously, without the intervention of a surgeon. One of Beth's wrists has fused in one place. 'It is not much different from wearing a splint,' she says. She says she would consider fusion as a treatment for her ankles if they got worse. Beth has also experienced a ruptured tendon in her arm. 'I was walking from the car with the keys in my hand, and suddenly I realized my thumb wasn't gripping them any more.' At the moment she has adjusted how she holds things with her left arm, but she hopes to have the tendon repaired by a surgeon sometime in the future.

Surgical operations for RA

If you really want the nitty-gritty on arthritis operations there is an excellent internet site offered by the US Arthritis Foundation which provides moving pictures and other useful detail. The reference is given in Useful addresses. This is just a brief round-up.

Arthroscopic surgery

An arthro*scope* ('scope' means 'look') is a device we have mentioned without naming it before. It is a thin fibre-optic probe inserted into the joint, usually under local anaesthetic, to investigate it visually or by retrieving small quantities of synovial tissue: a biopsy. It may be used by either expert rheumatologists or orthopaedic surgeons. Being able to see inside the joint enables the specialist to determine what aspect of the condition is causing problems. The biopsy can be used for diagnostic purposes or actually for the removal of damaged cartilage.

In recent years there have been major advances in what is known as key-hole surgery – carrying out remote-control work inside the body by means of a tiny incision and an arthroscope which enables the surgeon to see and operate remotely. The arthroscope is now used not only to remove internal parts of the joint (synovectomy) but to repair damaged or broken tendons and ligaments.

Synovectomy is one of the preventative procedures used by surgeons. A large portion of the inflamed joint lining (synovium) is removed to prevent it damaging the cartilage and eventually the bone of the joint. It is very effective at reducing the pain and swelling in the joint but it is not a permanent cure because the synovium may re-grow. In the past, synovectomy was carried out with open surgery. The use of key-hole surgery through the arthroscope has led to a greatly reduced recovery time from the operation.

Damaged tendons and ligaments are often repaired by connecting a separate but intact tendon to the ruptured one. The tendons most commonly affected are those that travel along the top of the hands down to the fingers.

Joint fusion

As we have seen from Beth's experience, bone fusion can occur when the connective tissues around the joint are so degraded that bone meets bone. Surgical fusion is performed on painful and unstable joints, usually those of the wrists, thumbs, feet or ankles. Fusion improves stability and reduces pain but it obviously applies permanent restriction to the joint. For this reason it is not suitable on the shoulder or hip joints, though it may be carried out on the neck joints of the spine.

Bone resection

Severe RA causes deformity by destroying the alignment of a joint. This can be improved by removing a small piece of bone (resecting) from one end of a joint. It is relatively simple and can be carried out on shoulders, elbows, wrists and feet to improve the range of movement in the joint and reduce pain. The procedure is done less frequently these days because joint replacement has advanced and is much more effective.

Joint replacement

There was a time when artificial implants were regarded with great suspicion. They were performed only in the elderly and less mobile who were less likely to wear out their expensive artificial joints.

But fashions in medicine change with advances in treatment, and nowadays old age is not automatically assumed to bring reduced function and physical decline. Maximum performance in later life is regarded as basic to good health and joint replacement is carried out sooner and more often with excellent results. Were it not for the high cost, there would probably be even more people walking around with artificial joints, principally knees and hips – the joints most frequently affected by OA.

RA patients constitute about one in ten of joint replacement subjects and they are more likely to require replacement elbow, wrist and ankle joints. These are available, but the outcome is not as predictable either for these delicate and complicated joints or for RA sufferers in general compared to those with OA. This is probably because they are suffering a systemic illness, and in addition many of the drugs they take reduce their physical resilience in one way or another.

There are many different sorts of joint prostheses and they are improving year on year. Some of the most recent, instead of using cement to connect the new joint to existing bone, provide a porous skeleton into which the patient's own bone can grow to weld the new joint in place. When successful, this kind of prosthesis is not only stronger and more durable but, in theory at least, less likely to need replacement in the future. The disadvantages include a longer period of rehabilitation while the natural bone infiltrates the prosthesis. The new bone growth may be less satisfactory in RA patients as a result of their illness and some of the medication they are prescribed.

Even the best joint replacement will not last for ever, which is why surgeons defer this solution until every other option has been tried. New techniques and materials have increased the life of a replacement to 15 years or more. But RA sufferers have other problems to deal with apart from the life of a replacement joint.

Complications of surgery

RA suffers are not straightforward candidates for surgery. They have an illness, and many of the medicines they take for that illness can affect the outcome of surgery. NSAIDs increase the risk of excessive bleeding and are usually stopped before an operation. Surgery is followed by a higher than normal risk of infection, including

---

Box 15   *RA survivors, Rick and Carol*

Rick is married to Carol. Their motto should be a version of the RAF's *Per ardua ad astra* – through adversity to the stars. Except that in their case the adversity was the road through RA. Rick calls their RA 'Arthur'. He and Arthur became acquainted on Rick's twenty-seventh birthday. He met Carol because of Arthur, through the internet, and Carol set up the first US arthritis website at About.com, run by RA sufferers to support other RA sufferers. (Details in Useful addresses.)

Complications of RA: you name it, Rick or Carol has had it, and yet they survived, dedicating their lives to helping other RA sufferers. In May 1998 Carol underwent her ninth arthritis-related surgical operation, a left ankle fusion. She had previously had both hips replaced and later revised, both knees replaced, and a right ankle fusion. 'A few months after the left ankle fusion Arthur gave us our first real scare,' writes Rick.

> The ankle became severely infected and Carol developed sepsis. She required ankle *debridement* [removal of damaged or infected tissue], a hospital stay, and several weeks of intravenous antibiotics at home to lead her to full recovery. In mid-2000 I had my right foot fused . . . A few weeks after surgery, this same foot developed a local infection requiring debridement, another hospital stay, and many months of antibiotics and wound care.

Rick's complications were not confined to those related to surgery.

> I began experiencing severe swelling and *oedema* [swelling caused by the kidneys being unable to clear fluid from the body] in my feet and legs I developed back and spine

---

exposure to resistant strains of bacteria which are associated with being in hospital, so drugs that inhibit the immune response – popular DMARDs like methotrexate and cyclosporine as well as the biologics – also have to be withdrawn. Even after withdrawal of these drugs, RA patients do not start on a level playing field where their immune systems are concerned and they are more likely than the average patient to suffer local infection after surgery. For this reason it is important to be sure that a patient has no minor infection

> problems and a critical general weakness took over. I began to lose my ability to walk . . . in hospital they discovered I had pericarditis [fluid and inflammation around the heart], a rare complication of rheumatoid arthritis. I was rushed into surgery to remove the fluid from my chest.

Rick's problems continued. The wound in his chest didn't heal; he developed an antibiotic-resistant infection – a problem for anyone who spends a lot of time in hospitals, and particularly RA patients whose medication undermines their auto-immune system. Rick spent months in hospital; his weight dropped to 185 pounds. He hallucinated and once or twice prepared himself for death.

But by April 2002 he was home again, for good.

> My wounds gradually healed, and I began extensive physical and occupational therapy to regain my function and mobility. I had cataract surgery to repair damage done by the high-dose steroids required during my long hospital stay. A successful wrist surgery followed too (synovectomy and tendon transfer). By late 2003, I took my first steps with a cane and some steps unassisted – a breakthrough from the platform walker I had been using.
>
> Carol and I have 45 years' experience between us of living and dealing with Arthur. We strive to be survivors of Arthur's many challenges and the striving never stops. We are marked by scars, literally and figuratively.

Rick and Carol's story illustrates one of the encouraging things about RA case histories. For many people a stay in hospital at death's door is the prelude to going though that door. Some RA sufferers approach the threshold, but come back.

– tooth decay or a bladder infection, for example – that might transfer its activity to the site of the surgery.

In spite of these provisos RA patients have a generally favourable experience of surgery. Even the smaller operations, like synovectomy, produce noticeable symptom relief, and people with RA learn to be thankful for small mercies. In the UK there is often quite a long wait for joint replacement. This has the effect of making the operation even more welcome when it materializes. For one couple's experience, see Box 15 on pp. 86–7.

Part 3: You and your future

11
Dealing with your feelings

Being ill makes anyone feel fed up. The realization that you are not only ill, and it hurts, and it's mucking up your life, but that it is also quite likely to go on for the rest of your life and in all probability it may even get worse, is a life-long prison sentence. No wonder when you learn you have RA you are more than fed up – you're wretched.

The problems are not only medical. Although the disease itself does not affect everyone who gets it in the same way, it is not too difficult to discuss the medical problems and how best to deal with them. Good medical treatment is based on broadly based, established protocols; this, that or the other drug, form of exercise, diet and behaviour is recommended by specialists who have studied their effectiveness in many patients. But there are practical, psychological, social and possibly even professional problems to be faced as well, which vary for each person even more than the course and nature of their disease.

In venturing into this territory even the professionals are on much less secure ground. One patient's problem may be that he hates asking for help; another that inflamed joints make it impossible for her to continue working as a dancer; another fears that her dependency and possible deformity will make it impossible ever to find a partner. Life circumstances and temperaments vary and call for different solutions to help people cope with illness, stress and change. How do you advise this heterogeneous group of individuals with their wide-ranging problems and repertoires of behaviour?

Facing up to the problem

There are no standard protocols or prescriptions for dealing with the psychological and social problems facing someone with RA. When you encounter depression and despair, loss of skill, an important job or a valued role as the strong, all-powerful provider there are no easy answers: there are only diffidently helpful suggestions of the 'You could try this; it helps some people' variety.

The first step in a coping campaign is to identify the enemy. When you develop RA you have to face up to some pretty unpleasant psychological companions: pain, fatigue, frustration, resentment, anger, despair, anxiety, fear and guilt, to name but a few of the furies that attend you. But there are weapons to combat them and allies to reinforce your efforts once you take a measure of the foe.

You are reading a book about this illness (your own or that of someone close to you). That is a step in the right direction. It implies that you want information, the first step towards taking charge and overcoming those demons. People do not all face the same ones. One person is overcome by rage, another with helpless despair. Perhaps you don't have any problem with moods – see Beth's example below – but skim through the chapter anyway. You may already be doing some of the things we suggest. Good for you. You may also discover insight into how others feel even if it isn't your problem.

Different reactions to the RA diagnosis

Consider three RA patients we have already met and the contrasting ways they responded to being diagnosed. Christine – the one who fought the post-code lottery and got her infliximab – is obviously a fighter.

> I can remember the day I was diagnosed. It was a very chilly spring evening and, after several blood tests, my doctor just looked at me and said; 'You have RA and there is no cure for it.' I walked out of the surgery in a daze, knowing that the pain and the stiffness that had been coming on for a year were never going to go away. I cried just once and decided I was going to fight it.

Beth, whose mother had RA before her, has constructed a life which keeps her RA private.

> I suppose I have dealt with it by ignoring it as much as possible. Yes, I was obviously depressed when I realized I had RA. I had to

give up all idea of becoming a 'cellist. But I decided it wasn't going to stop me doing anything else I cared about. I dropped out of college in Australia, where I lived at that time, came to England, got married, started a family, found a different career that didn't require agile fingers. I don't tell people I have RA and usually they don't realize.

Contrast this attitude with Lisa's (Chapter 8). Perhaps Lisa's arthritis was worse than Beth's; perhaps she was just a different sort of personality; but Lisa is not alone in that she has professionalized coping with RA and is now advising others how to do the same. Lisa is no exception. Carol (Chapter 10) also advises others. She met her husband, Rick, another RA sufferer, through an arthritis chatroom she was running on America Online. Both their lives are now focused on helping others with the disease. To some extent RA has *become* their lives.

But then look at Dorothy (Chapter 5), who was prone to depression even before she got RA. RA made her so tired she sometimes refused to get out of bed for days. That made her symptoms worse and she added guilt to fatigue because she knew she was neglecting her family. For nearly a year Dorothy virtually shut down her life. She hardly went out, to take the children to and from school or to meet friends – shopping she found impossible because she couldn't lift anything, or manage the pedals on the car. But then Dorothy discovered one of the many arthritis self-help groups on the internet. She started talking to other sufferers; she heard how they dealt with fatigue, with feeling a failure, with having no energy for the exercise they knew they should do. Dorothy had discovered someone who didn't just say 'Poor you,' but who suggested 'Why don't you . . . ?' when she described her problems. She wanted to meet other RA sufferers, which made her want to drive, and that was important enough for her to do her exercises so that she could drive comfortably. Through meeting others Dorothy learned new ways of viewing her circumstances. She felt less helpless and more motivated to do something to improve her life.

Talk to someone

Most of the unpleasant emotions that plague people with a chronic illness are better out than in. By acknowledging and talking about feelings you get a handle on them, and hopefully you may change them for the better. If you are an articulate person you start at an advantage. You probably already have family, friends or colleagues with whom you discuss things. When you are depressed you know which friend can cheer you up, when you are angry which one will calm you down. If you are not good at expressing your feelings, talking about them requires more effort. A trained therapist or counsellor can encourage you to look inward and analyse what troubles you with a view to achieving a more positive state of mind.

One of the advantages of talking to professionals – not necessarily doctors, but those experienced in assessing psychological problems – is that they are able to judge whether your depression or anxiety is serious enough to be treated with drugs. It is perfectly reasonable to feel such emotions when you first have RA. Let's face it, you have something to be depressed about. But however justified, depression is something best overcome. It makes the other things we have to deal with worse. Taking a drug that makes you feel less anxious (an *anxiolytic*) or less depressed (an *antidepressant*) is quite a reasonable step provided you regard it as a temporary solution, a breathing space to come to terms and start adopting more positive attitudes. Such drugs are not a long-term solution to coping with chronic illness.

If there is a counsellor attached to your GP's practice, she may be able to help. If not, both the National Rheumatoid Arthritis Society and Arthritis Care have helplines and a list of local support groups in the UK. The Arthritis Foundation and a number of other organizations do the same in the USA. (See Useful addresses.)

Dealing with depression

Anyone who has ever been depressed recognizes the symptoms. Nothing seems worth doing; nothing interests you, nothing gives you pleasure. Even when the sun shines you feel gloomy, and if it rains – oh Gawd! You can't sleep for thinking about awful things. You can't eat because food seems pointless and tasteless.

An experienced counsellor first offers you a chance to unburden yourself, listening and showing understanding. But rehearsing negative feelings does not change them. She will suggest alternative ways of thinking, feeling and behaving tailored to your particular situation and concerns. If you are lucky you may have friends or family who can do this.

Don't cut yourself off from others

Which 'others' only you know. Keep doing things with the children; keep going to church or to the football matches; keep singing with the choir, visiting friends, having your parents to lunch. Keep walking your dog or feeding the wild birds. Animals don't notice if you are not quite as nimble as you were, and those who know you make allowances. Being with others opens the door for you to focus on other people and activities, something other than your own disrupted life. Doing things you are used to or things you are good at establishes continuity that counteracts those feelings of disruption and loss. When you switch the spotlight away from yourself, perhaps to help someone else or to solve a shared problem, you stop being a victim and become an actor in life again. And being an actor restores your self-esteem.

Give yourself rewards

Make a list of things you enjoy. It's difficult when you are low, and to start with you may have to enlist help. 'Remember how much you laughed at *Monsieur Hulot's Holiday*?' says your partner. Go out and get the video. Laughter is therapeutic. Write down favourite pieces of music, favourite foods, places in the country, the seaside, the warm feeling of caring for young animals. With luck you will find some rewards you can keep on hand to lift your spirits when you are down. Something that makes you laugh is particularly useful, or something sensual, like stroking a cat, a rabbit or a fur coat.

Not all the things that give you pleasure will be easily accessible but listing them is a valuable exercise in itself. It turns your attention towards positive, enjoyable experiences. With practice you can train yourself to *think* about good experiences as a way of driving out negative thoughts, especially if they keep you awake. If you have a good imagination you may be able to conjure up lying on a beach in the sun, or hearing the sound of the nightingale when you want to go to sleep. If you can't imagine it, get yourself a soothing sounds tape to send you off.

Accentuate the positive

There is always a different way of interpreting things. If a negative thought comes to you, turn it round as though you were arguing with someone. 'I so miss playing the 'cello,' becomes: 'Having played the 'cello makes me enjoy hearing it played well.' 'I'm such a burden on everyone,' becomes: 'I'm so lucky that everyone is so helpful.' 'Lifting things has become such a hassle,' becomes: 'I'm getting pretty nifty at finding ways of lifting that don't hurt my joints.' Again, to begin with it will probably help if you can start the argument with someone else, counsellor, partner or friend. Once you get the idea, every negative thought becomes a challenge: how can I turn it into a positive one?

Carol worked to convert a sense of loss into one of transformation. 'The loss was slow, just like the progression of the disease,' she says.

> Aspects of my life that I had carved out for years were being taken away from me. There seemed to be a slow erosion of my life taking place directly proportional to the erosion of my joints ... I needed the mental changes to correlate with the physical changes. I wasn't really disappearing, but I was changing ... The focus had to shift from what I had lost to what I still had.

Finding the positive interpretation to the negatives in your life is also the key to increasing your self-esteem. The reasoning goes: people with RA find things difficult, they suffer pain and fatigue. It follows that by meeting this challenge and overcoming the difficulties people with RA are fantastically courageous, resourceful, determined, ingenious and in every way admirable. Just you believe it.

Do something for others

This is not a pious admonition. It's an established, observable phenomenon that if you start to think about others, or busy yourself doing things for them, you worry less about yourself and you feel better about your own situation. The second half is obvious: people who care for others are good people, useful, needed. The first half works by replacing inward-turned anxieties with positive concerns and actions.

Exercise

It's a well-known fact, experienced by athletes and those who exercise for less urgent reasons than because they have RA, that exercise gives you a natural high. Some people become addicted to it, exercise to achieve it and feel down if they can't. The explanation is thought to be that exercise releases natural body chemicals called *endorphins*. These appear to reduce pain and generally to lift the spirits. Exercise also concentrates the mind because it involves effort. Unpleasant, intrusive thoughts recede. Your whole mind and body become focused on the present. Those who don't exercise are sceptical. Get into your exercise routine and discover the truth.

Professional counsellors and other RA sufferers will have other tips to offer. This is just a beginning. We started with depression because this is the most widespread emotional problem in RA. Some of the techniques for combating depression will also help with other negative feelings.

Dealing with anxiety and stress

Anxiety and stress are not the same thing but they often go together. Or, more precisely, the one leads to the other. Anxiety and fear – the former a generalized, unfocused form of the latter – are, like depression, understandable and justified in anyone with RA, a condition that is full of uncertainty. They are nevertheless unhelpful feelings. Someone inclined to pessimism encounters uncertainty and becomes anxious about unspecified awfulness and fearful about the known bad outcomes that are possible. 'I shall be confined to a wheel-chair; I'll never play tennis again; I won't be able to carry the baby; no one will find me attractive . . .' But the optimist sees in uncertainty the possibility that the worst *may not* happen. There are clear advantages in aiming for optimism.

Teach yourself optimism by accessing the facts. Only 5 per cent of RA sufferers experience the seriously debilitating manifestations of the disease. Even among them it is not necessarily permanent. (See Rick's story in Chapter 10.) Seventy-five per cent of RA sufferers continue with their normal lives; a large proportion experience some interruption in the progress of the disease thanks to drugs. Understanding and treatment for RA is progressing by leaps and bounds. (See Chapter 13.) A cure may even come in your lifetime. And something Beth mentions: 'Taking all those pain-killers, you are never going to have a headache ever again!'

If anxiety leads on to stress, a whole host of unpleasant consequences can arise. Stress leads to tension, leads to increased pain, leads to lowered resistance to infection and a general reduction in your immune response. If you do feel stressed it is important to resolve it. Again, identifying the enemy is the number one goal. Stress often hinges on a particular situation. It may build up whenever you face a particular task or social occasion. If you can identify the precipitating cause, then you can negotiate a way round it. You feel stressed whenever you meet your mother-in-law because she goes on and on about your illness and how frightful it is. Get your husband to tell her to change her tune or you won't be able to meet her. You are stressed when picking up the toddler from nursery school because you have problems lifting him into the car. Make friends with another mother or a teacher and ask for assistance. They will be only too glad and he will soon be fastening himself into his own seat-belt.

There is nothing noble about enduring stressful situations; modify them or avoid them. If they are unavoidable – getting through a long working day can be like this – work out a compromise: take short breaks; go somewhere quiet for a few minutes. At home have a hot bath, sit quietly and listen to soothing music. Take time to unwind and gather your resources. If it means negotiation with an employer, do it in the confidence that compromise is a constructive solution.

Formal techniques that combat stress and relieve tension include muscle relaxation. This is like isometric exercise. It involves getting into a comfortable position – not necessarily lying down – in a quiet place, closing your eyes and gradually working through all the muscle groups in your body, from the toes to the scalp: first clenching; then relaxing and feeling the difference; then maintaining the relaxed state. You have to put a little thought into how you group your muscles: toes, ankles, calves, knees, thighs. But by the time you have got to your pelvis the magic will begin to work. Dr Edmund Jacobson, who first described the technique in 1929, claimed that it was literally impossible to feel nervous or anxious if all your muscles were perfectly relaxed. It takes practice, but it pays off.

Another technique of which there are many varieties is meditation. You usually meditate by focusing your mind on a single, soothing thing: a beautiful word – say 'serendipity'; a beautiful sound – a blackbird's song; a visual image like waves breaking on the sea-shore; or simply your own breathing. It takes practice, like muscle relaxation. To begin with you can actually say the word to yourself over and over again – what is called a mantra. If you are concentrating on your breathing, one technique is to breathe in deeply to a short count (1 to 4), hold for a few seconds, and then exhale to a slow count (5 to 12). Practise making the exhale slower and longer without strain. Again, it is the act of mental concentration that gradually clears all unpleasant thoughts from your mind. But the controlled breathing also calms you, slowing down your pulse and heart-rate. It is an excellent way to go to sleep and may be the origin of counting sheep.

Dealing with anger and resentment

It is not so obvious that someone with RA should feel anger. Not everyone does. Most people are either sorry for themselves or angry with others when misfortune strikes. But these two emotions are closer than you think.

Have you ever thought, 'Why me? What did I do to deserve this?'? Have you felt that life is unjust? It is quite natural to look for something to blame when bad things happen to you. And when there really isn't anyone or anything it is almost worse. Resentment is left flailing around wildly and the innocent are as likcly to be hurt as the non-existent guilty. Some people turn against their doctors because they are helpless and treatment so slow or ineffective. Others turn against employers or work colleagues, who don't understand the problems they have to cope with, or against their family, either because they don't realize that the most mundane domestic tasks now require a superhuman effort or, conversely, because they start to treat you like an invalid and that makes you feel one. It's impossible do the right thing for someone who is angry. And suppressed anger is the most difficult thing to deal with. 'Rage, rage against the dying of the light,' said the poet Dylan Thomas. Get suppressed anger out into the light; put your feelings into words as a start. If you give voice to your justifiable rage against fate for dealing you the RA card, hopefully your close friends and family will sympathize and understand. If they don't, then rage to your therapist. But having raged, move on. 'Been there, seen that, got the Rage T-shirt.' Anger is energy; use it to solve or circumvent the situations that prompt it.

Negotiate a work schedule that gives you the opportunity for a break now and then; ask your family to lend a hand with the things you find most difficult, or ask them to let you do it in your own way and in your own time, without comment, please.

Try to scale down your expectations. You are now someone coping with a chronic disease. That leaves less room for other things, or means other things take longer. One way to make your expectations of yourself more realistic is to do everything little by little or a day at a time. 'Tomorrow I will walk to get the newspaper.' Or, if that turns out to be hard work: 'Tomorrow I will walk to the corner and back.' Only do the longer distance when the shorter becomes easy. And if and when you manage to build upon what you undertake, congratulate yourself. For someone with RA even small achievements warrant a medal.

Difficulty with special relationships

There are particular problems to be faced in dealing with people who depend on you: children, but also partners and parents. How do you rearrange the job of reliable prop to that of someone who also needs support? The first thing to do is to dismiss guilt. Tell yourself firmly that you have nothing to feel guilty about. No one is to blame for you getting RA, let alone you. The situation has to be dealt with, by you and by everyone involved with you. People who value you will not mind making adjustments.

But if you are the sort of person on whom others rely, much of your self-esteem may depend on the role. RA requires that you give up some of this central importance. Just as you got gratification from being needed so, by requiring others to help and support you, you are actually giving them importance and a chance to be responsible and caring towards you. Nothing is more generous than to allow others to give to you. Remember Beth bringing back books from the library for her mother, buying her own school uniform? Maybe this early experience of being adult and responsible bolstered her self-esteem and helped her deal with RA at first hand.

So ask for help; show warmth and appreciation when it comes and be understanding when it cannot be provided. You are free to ask when you need help as long as they feel free to say when they cannot provide it.

A problem with children is maintaining their routine. Children like to know what will happen and when, in a regular pattern. But

RA makes it difficult to be reliable because you cannot be sure whether you have a good or a bad day ahead of you. You will need to accustom children to some degree of unreliability. It's not bad practice for the life ahead. 'I'm sorry, Jake, I won't be able to collect you from swimming today. My RA is bad. I've asked Tim's mother to bring you home. I'll be there another time.' For this reason it is as well not to make promises, just in case you can't keep them. Instead, start a programme of nice surprises. 'Hey guys, I'm feeling pretty fit today, shall we go to the sea with a picnic?'

Not forgetting sex

Partnerships are based on reciprocity – the mutually agreed complementary exchange of love, confidence and care. When one of you becomes sick the balance is skewed. You have to re-negotiate who gives what and who receives. There is a risk that this new factor will aggravate any conflict between a couple. If one of you feels put upon by the other, RA will make it worse, whether you are the sufferer or the partner who has to pick up the reins dropped by the other. If one of you has been more enthusiastic about sex than the other, RA can easily be made an excuse to withdraw, on either side. And even someone with a previously healthy appetite may find RA causes it to flag. All sorts of anxieties come flooding in. The person with the RA feels unattractive because they are ill and physically restricted. Pain gets in the way of pleasure. His or her partner worries about doing something that adds to the pain. And stiff, painful hip or knee joints are a direct physical obstruction to traditional positions for sexual intercourse.

The problem affects two people. Solving it requires discussion – between partners, and if communication on the subject is difficult, with a professional counsellor. It may require some renegotiation of what is comfortable and pleasurable. Dr Jackson Rainer of Webb University in the USA writing on the Enliven advice line (run by the manufacturers of etanercept), recommends rediscovering intimacy through talk and touch rather than going straight to intercourse. 'The biggest sex organ is the skin and the best sex organ is the brain,' he says. He advises using what sex therapists call the *sensate focus.* This is a technique that recalls the love-making of beginners; you try to give pleasure through sensual, sexy touching and arousing words and hold back on penetration. The restraint is said to rekindle desire and ensure that when intercourse finally takes place, at a time when both parties are equally ready for it, it is more fulfilling.

Rediscovering the tentative, exploratory behaviour of young lovers is good therapy for old couples even if one of them hasn't got RA. But there are occasionally more fundamental problems than stiff, painful joints. The side effects of some RA medication may affect desire, and some men with RA have reported problems with getting an erection. If this is traced to low levels of the male hormone androgen it can be treated by male hormone replacement therapy. Women RA sufferers are more likely to have problems related to body-image; they just don't feel sexy or feminine any more.

If you and your partner have problems like these do seek help. RA is bad enough without letting it take other pleasures away from you. Your GP or the arthritis support organizations listed at the end of this book can recommend a specialist clinic or skilled counsellors.

12

Modifying your life-style

How much should you change your life-style because you have RA? This is principally a personal decision – what life activities do you undertake that will be hampered by sore, restricted joints? – but it is also subject to medical fashion. Fifty or even twenty years ago, books on coping with arthritis (OA as well as RA) were full of illustrations of special tools for opening jars, special bars for pulling yourself out of baths, swivel seats for getting you out of cars and long-handled grippers for picking things off the floor. The catalogues are still around and a visit to the internet will offer you endless clever devices that you can spend money on if you enjoy such things or feel a genuine personal need. (Some are listed in Box 16 on p. 104.) But the professional advice these days is more likely to be: 'Use as little special equipment as possible because some of it actually interferes with your ability to function independently, especially if you come to rely upon it too heavily.'

If you find you do need help in some physical manoeuvre because your joints are being unco-operative, it is probably better to make use of something you already have lying about. 'My mother used to swear by an adjustable spanner for opening things,' says Beth. 'I myself favour a pair of nut-crackers.'

No tool is better than common sense

That said, you have a disease that affects some of the most used joints in the body. It would be foolhardy to think you could ignore it completely. What most RA patients report is that they instinctively become more aware of the limitations of their affected joints. It becomes second nature to adopt protective or supportive ways of doing things. For example, you turn the cap on a new jar of marmalade. You feel the strain on your knuckles; you can see them being pushed back, towards the little finger. Puncture the lid and go for the nut-crackers. 'If it feels as though it's damaging my joints, it probably will. So I find another way,' says Beth. You lift a kettle full of water: automatically you will feel the need of two hands to limit strain on the wrists. You lift a tray: two hands underneath rather than one each side putting strain on the wrists. Heavy shopping? Get a basket on wheels. Should you drive an automatic to save strain on the ankles? 'I suppose you should,' says Beth, 'but I've never got round to it. I just adjust the way I drive.'

Techniques, which you may find yourself adopting instinctively, are outlined in booklets supplied by the Arthritis Research Campaign (ARC) in the UK and support organizations all over the world. They are part of natural joint protection. The guidelines are:

- take notice of pain – it serves as a warning;
- spread the load over several joints;
- use larger, stronger joints;
- use less effort;
- avoid positions which push your joints towards deformity;
- avoid gripping things tightly;
- use your joints in more stable positions.

Protecting your joints reduces the risk of developing deformities.

A simple device that almost everyone recommends is the joint splint. You can make this yourself (see Figure 7 opposite) or buy one from a supplier of medical equipment or a pharmacy. A resting splint is worn when you are resting or sleeping. It consists of a smooth, rigid support beneath the joint, secured by straps or bands in a couple of places either side so that it is held firmly in position. An elastic splint for the wrist provides support without immobility while you are working. Wearing one encourages you to adopt handling techniques that do not strain the wrist.

Research shows that if you can adopt joint protection methods you will suffer less pain and find everyday domestic tasks easier. People who use them, especially combined with a regular exercise programme, also have less morning stiffness and fewer flare-ups of their RA.

But the professional can also help

Many people with RA adapt their life-style simply by reading helpful literature and using their own common sense, but specialist help is usually available at the rheumatology departments of

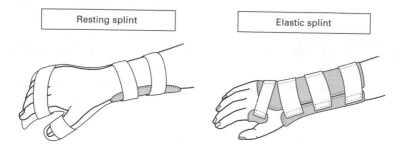

Figure 7 Two types of splint

hospitals. An occupational therapist can advise on modifying your domestic routine and adopting joint protection procedures. Some departments run training programmes for groups of RA patients who help each other as well as learning from the therapists.

Beth's mother, whose RA is more advanced and dates from a time when there was less disease-modifying treatment available, has several useful household aids. She lives on a single level to avoid having to negotiate stairs, she has had a ramp fitted outside the back door, so that those days she feels like sticking to her wheel-chair she can get in and out without having to go up the front-door steps, and she has had a key 'pad' fitted in place of a lock because using keys was becoming difficult. Beth describes a customized 'walker' made of a frame with wheels at the front which they have adapted to take a basket and a child-seat. 'Considering all the years she was bedridden it's a great sight to see her go down to the shops pushing the walker with her two-year-old grandchild in the chair and the dog on a lead,' says Beth.

What about diet?

Beware of putting too much emphasis on the role of food in illness. The phrase 'You are what you eat' is a wild exaggeration and has many delusions to answer for. Yes, it is possible to make yourself less healthy by eating too much of the wrong things or too little of the right, but with few exceptions – genuine, relatively rare allergies or intolerances – food is neither the cause of disease nor a cure for it.

You will nevertheless be bombarded by books, magazine articles and sites on the internet that promise instant response from the introduction or removal of some dietary element quite possibly costing you big money. Take all with a very large metaphorical pinch of salt. (Don't take too much real salt because that could be bad for your blood pressure.) People can be very passionate about food, and if you believe that one food is making you feel better or another causing you flare-ups it will do no harm to follow your instinct. Remember, however, that only DMARDs and biologic medicines have been scientifically proved to have any effect on the progress of RA.

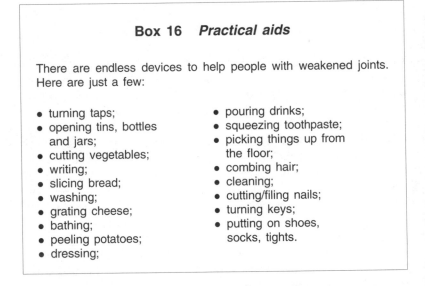

Box 16 *Practical aids*

There are endless devices to help people with weakened joints. Here are just a few:

- turning taps;
- opening tins, bottles and jars;
- cutting vegetables;
- writing;
- slicing bread;
- washing;
- grating cheese;
- bathing;
- peeling potatoes;
- dressing;

- pouring drinks;
- squeezing toothpaste;
- picking things up from the floor;
- combing hair;
- cleaning;
- cutting/filing nails;
- turning keys;
- putting on shoes, socks, tights.

It is important that you eat well if you have RA and that you avoid putting on weight. Since your exercise regime is unlikely to be of sufficient vigour – at least to begin with – to encourage weight loss, you will have to control your weight by eating the right quantities of the right food. There are plenty of places to find out about a healthy diet: it contains moderate amounts of protein, not missing out on fish, plenty of fruit and vegetables, high-fibre grains and cereals and moderate amounts of fat, especially saturated (dairy) fats, and certain components – vitamins and trace elements – which will automatically be present if you get the balance right. Here is not the place to go into details.

When it comes to affecting your illness, there is *some* evidence that *some* people are sensitive to certain foods and that these foods may aggravate their symptoms. Obviously, if you think you have identified such a culprit you should avoid it, though check it out with the medical team before you deny yourself something central to your diet like bread or milk. People who have an intolerance of certain foods – *gluten* as present in wheat cereals and the common additive monosodium glutamate are both well documented – may find these also aggravate their symptoms, but they should be avoiding them anyway by virtue of their intolerance.

There is also a hypothesis that foods which have *antioxidant* and anti-inflammatory properties may lessen the symptoms of RA. Cod-liver oil, other fish oils and evening primrose oil have been shown to have a mild effect on the pain and swelling of RA. It is thought that the latest star in the nutrition galaxy, the fatty acid omega-3, present in fish oils which are also rich in vitamin D, may have anti-inflammatory properties. Studies support the idea that vitamin D, which is obtainable partly from sunlight and cold-water fish, and which the body needs to absorb calcium, might have a protective role in RA. It is clearly important to reduce the osteoporosis which is a side effect of using corticosteroids. However, no vitamin supplement has been demonstrated to reduce the structural damage caused by RA.

Are there any alternatives?

Alternative cures for RA are certainly on offer, in their thousands, but there is little scientific evidence that they have any effect on either the symptoms or the progress of RA. Some treatments may be 'complementary', but there is really no 'alternative' to NSAID and DMARD therapy. Wherever there is a chronic illness affecting many people which is inadequately controlled by orthodox medicine you will find the mushroom growth of alternative cures. It represents the capitalist marketing instinct responding to a natural human desire to try any port in a storm.

Sadly, the most that can be said of most alternative remedies proposed for RA is that some – massage or aromatherapy, for example – are soothing, relaxing and/or psychologically beneficial. Others, like homeopathy, do no harm but do no apparent good either.

Some herbal remedies may actually interfere with anti-rheumatic medication and a number of so-called traditional medicines, especially Chinese remedies, have been found to contain large quantities of steroids and other active drugs. The problem with most of these medicines, many of which do certainly contain active ingredients, is that there is no standardized way of manufacturing them that will guarantee which ingredients they contain and how much. Unlike licensed drugs, they are not required to go through rigorous clinical testing procedures, there is no way of knowing what, if anything, is in them, what, if anything, may be their effects on which particular sub-group of sick people or whether they will interact with other medicines. The word 'natural', often used for such cures, is little more than a word used on the label.

Maintain your general health to minimize RA

Look back on our discussion of how to treat and beat RA. With the exception of the drugs, which although they help control RA may have unpleasant side effects upon the rest of your body, all the advice is what any expert would recommend to the general population to maintain health into old age. The exercise regime – start gently and build up to maintain maximum performance not only in affected joints but your whole body; the psychological advice – talk about your problems, resolve stress, find a way round obstacles, be realistic in your expectations and enjoy life; the dietary advice – do not get overweight, eat a balanced diet. Even the advice to protect your joints by small modifications of behaviour and the tools you use is good advice for anyone dealing with ageing joints and muscles.

The way to survive RA turns out to be to utilize the knowledge of modern medicine, keep healthy and get the most out of all that life still offers you. In Carol's words,

The new life I was living was bound by limitations but it was not a bad life, just different. There was a need to alter certain goals and dreams and develop new ones. There was a need to adapt daily routines and long-term plans. There still is much pleasure and happiness to be squeezed out of life. The loss of oneself is really just a rebirth.

13

Hope for the future

The medical research community is cautious about promising new cures. Giant strides in the understanding of what causes disease are one thing: the development and testing of treatments based on new understanding takes at least ten years. Many are the hopeful young drugs that fall by the wayside in that time.

But where RA is concerned there is encouraging movement on many fronts, from the genetic basis of why some people are susceptible to RA, through the triggers in the environment that may set it off, to the functioning of the immune system and why it goes wrong in illnesses like diabetes and RA, to how to interrupt the destructive cascade of inflammation at any one of a number of points.

Understanding who gets RA and why

Twelve centres around the USA are collaborating to study the genes of 1,000 families in which two or more siblings have RA. This work is being organized by the North American Rheumatoid Arthritis Consortium (NARAC). The hope is that small differences in the genetic make-up of family members who do develop the disease and those who don't may make it possible to predict vulnerable people in the future. If such genes could be identified it might also be possible to alter them (gene therapy), although this form of therapy is still in the experimental stage even for those illnesses, like the bleeding disorder haemophilia, where the culprit gene has been identified.

More is being learned about the genetic basis for RA susceptibility by studying rats which have an auto-immune inflammatory arthritis that resembles RA. Much important work in understanding disease processes goes on in animals. Without it new cures would be impossible. There are striking similarities between rats and humans, and some genetic regions that affect both susceptibility and severity in animals have already been identified.

The role of hormones in RA

Why do so many more women than men get RA? Scientists have long proposed that the sex hormones and other ways in which men and women differ may contribute to differences in their immune response and hence to their susceptibility to RA. There is a complex relationship between the hormones, the nervous and the immune systems in RA, and it is possible that changes in the levels of steroid hormones like oestrogen and testosterone during the lifetime might be related to the development of RA and to improvements or flare-ups in the disease. For example, scientists have long wondered why it is that RA often improves during pregnancy. One study suggests that this may be because a woman carrying a child in the womb produces special proteins that enable her immune system to distinguish between the cells of her own body and those of the baby, which are in some ways 'foreign', without rejecting it as an invader. If a pregnant woman's immune system becomes subtly different in the way it differentiates 'self' and 'other', it might be possible to capitalize on this natural occurrence to develop new treatments for RA.

Understanding the triggers for RA

If we understood what lights the spark of RA could we do something to protect people from it? Some researchers believe the incidence of RA may be less now than it was in history and they hypothesize that this could be because modern hygiene and vaccines protect present-day populations from many of the infections that were endemic to past civilizations. There is certainly a growing body of evidence that some infectious agent, a virus or bacterium, acts as the trigger in those who have inherited a predisposition to RA. Scientists are trying to identify what these might be and also to understand the mechanism by which a healthy reaction by the immune system in repelling such an agent changes into the unhealthy immune reaction of RA. Understanding the interaction of the trigger and the immune system could lead to new therapies.

Finding out what goes wrong in the immune system

Understanding of the complexities of the immune system and how it sometimes malfunctions is advancing on several fronts. The Arthritis Research Campaign supports more than 60 units all over the UK following many different lines of inquiry. Blocking other inflammatory cytokines in addition to TNF and IL-1 is being investigated using naturally occurring soluble receptors (see Box 17) or specially engineered MoAbs. Researchers are focusing on other interleukins (they number from IL-1 to IL-18) that damp down inflammation. At Northwestern University in the USA researchers successfully introduced a gene that codes for one of these anti-inflammatory cytokines (IL-13) into mice and achieved a reduction in the production of pro-inflammatory cytokines.

Several British teams have as their goal re-balancing the effect of

---

Box 17 *Partial blockade of cytokine IL-6 studied at Cardiff*

One of the limitations of otherwise effective biologic agents that target pro-inflammatory cytokines is the side effect that patients become extremely vulnerable to infection, specifically tuberculosis. Another is that 30 per cent of patients receiving anti-TNF therapies fail to respond to treatment. New strategies targeting other pro-inflammatory cytokines are therefore essential. The pro-inflammatory cytokine IL-6 is already the target of one new drug in the pipeline (see 'New drugs in the pipeline and old ones put to new use'). A team at Cardiff University has discovered that IL-6 has a key role in the transformation of the normal, innate immune response (which dies down when the invader is vanquished) and the pathological, acquired immune response which promotes a chronic inflammatory state. In RA, IL-6's co-ordinating function becomes disrupted. In an inflamed joint the pro-inflammation messages from IL-6 are received by a soluble receptor, and targeting this receptor suppresses joint inflammation and associated tissue damage. The team has managed to block this receptor, not with an engineered MoAb but with an antagonist that occurs naturally in the circulation, a signalling protein they call sgp130. Therapeutic administration of sgp130 would simply supplement existing sgp130 concentrations to achieve its desired effect. Since sgp130 specifically targets only the receptors in the inflamed joint, the benign activity of IL-6 would remain unaffected. The team hope that partial blockade of IL-6 activity may be sufficient to re-balance the inflammatory response without significantly disrupting the body's normal defence mechanisms.

various cytokines to achieve reduced inflammation in the joint without damaging the immune system's capacity to defend the body from infection. Other groups are looking at the premature ageing of RA T cells and their failure to go through the normal process of *apoptosis* (programmed cell death) when there is nothing left to attack (see Box 18).

Box 18 *'Elderly' RA T cells studied at Birmingham?*

One way in which the immune system of RA patients differs from that of other people is that it responds poorly to normal challenges, making them more vulnerable to infection. At the University of Birmingham, UK, they are looking at differences in RA T lymphocytes that might explain this. Instead of undergoing the natural process of apoptosis these cells keep going in an 'elderly' state, continuing to drive the production of inflammatory cytokines like TNF inside the joint. Cell ageing is thought to be connected to increasing numbers of reactive oxygen molecules, known as free radicals, building up in the body and altering the function of lymphocytes. These damaging chemicals are normally mopped up by good chemicals called antioxidants present in fruit, vegetable and other foods rich in vitamin C. Some of these are only present at low levels in RA patients. This ties up with a finding that a deficiency of vitamin C in the diet makes people more prone to arthritis.

Gene therapy

At Barts and the London Hospital in London they are experimenting with a sophisticated form of gene therapy whereby the patient's own cells are altered to produce the kind of therapeutic protein used in biologic treatments that correct the balance of pro-inflammatory and anti-inflammatory cytokines. The hope is that the genes could be made to act inside the affected joints in response to the challenge of an RA flare-up. And in the University of East Anglia they are also experimenting with gene therapy that will enable joints to produce their own natural inhibitors to check the destructive enzymes that attack cartilage and bone in the advanced stages of RA.

Bone loss and bone growth

At Aberdeen they are investigating why osteoclasts (the bone-absorbing cells) keep going in RA rather than embracing apoptosis as they do in healthy joints, and at the Royal Veterinary College in London they are investigating ways of promoting bone growth that could be helpful in RA.

New drugs in the pipeline and old ones put to new use

A number of new drugs, combinations of drugs or improvements on drugs are in the pipeline. New biologics, based on naturally occurring body chemicals and designed to interrupt the inflammation cascade, are in development. One that uses a MoAb (Atlizumab) that blocks IL-6 is in the early stages of clinical trials and has shown favourable results, with no evidence of toxicity or increased incidence of infection.

New combinations of drugs are always being tried. A member of the tetracycline family, an antibiotic called doxycycline which has been around for some time, has been shown to improve on the effect of methotrexate on its own.

On the dietary front it has been confirmed that the latest star in the nutritional firmament, omega-3, a fatty acid found in cold-water fish and some plant-seed oils, reduces the inflammation of RA, though tolerating the vast quantities of the oil necessary to obtain the effect may be something some stomachs may balk at.

A small study reported recently in *The Lancet* (116 patients over only six months) concluded that the anti-cholesterol drugs known as statins had an anti-inflammatory effect in RA patients as well as preventing cardiovascular disease.

And in the clinic

Less glamorous but nevertheless highly valuable research goes on at the level of disease management. At the level of quality of life (those all-important 'qualys') studies have confirmed what therapists and patients already knew intuitively: quite small improvements in a patient's sense of physical and mental well-being can have an impact on the progress of RA and on the success of health-care services.

Evidence-based research like this emphasizes the practical value of psychological as well as pharmacological treatment, and enables health-care teams to plan treatment programmes for the here and now, rather than in some idealized future.

Glossary

Acetylsalicylic acid   aspirin's chemical name

Aerobic exercise   exercise that demands increased lung capacity

Aichmophobia or Belonephobia   an abnormal fear of needles or sharp objects

Anaemia   a shortage of oxygen-bearing red blood cells

Ankylosing spondylitis   an inflammatory condition of the spine

Antibodies   specialized cells produced by the body to fight foreign invaders: viruses or bacteria

Antidepressants   drugs that counter depression

Antigen   something foreign that stimulates antibodies to attack

Antioxidant   a vitamin, mineral or other organic substance that mops up highly reactive oxygen molecules that cause damage in the body (free radicals)

Anxiolytic   drugs that counter anxiety

Arthritis   inflammation of the joints

Arthropathy   disease of the joints

Arthroscope   a thin fibre-optic probe for investigating the interior of joints

Aspirate   to suck out

Atrophy   to wither away, shrink

Auto-immune disease   one in which the body's natural defence mechanisms are turned against its own tissues

Biologic medicines   medicines that mimic processes that occur naturally in the body

Biopsy   a small sample of living tissue taken to do laboratory tests

Bursa   a protective cushion full of fluid that pads pressure points in a mobile joint

Cardiovascular exercise   the kind of exercise that develops the capacity of the heart and lungs

Carpal tunnel   a narrow passage under the wrist through which tendons and nerves pass from the arm to the palm of the hand and which can become inflamed

Cartilage   the tough, smooth lining which coats the moving surface of joints; gristle

113

Chronic   coming and going; off and on; as opposed to acute – unremitting

Clavicles   the collar-bones (under the top shirt button)

Cognitive behaviour therapy   learning to change attitudes and the way you think

Colitic arthritis   arthritis affecting the lining of the colon

Collagen   a protein which is the principal component of connective tissue; bundled together in elastic-like ropes, it loses its elasticity with age

Colon   the lower bowel leading to the rectum

Cortisone/corticosteroids   naturally occurring hormones or drugs modelled on them that reduce inflammation, among other things

Cyclo-oxygenase (COX)   enzymes that stimulate the production of prostaglandins and which are the focus of new, improved pain-killers

Cytokines   chemical messengers that communicate between cells

Debridement   surgical removal of dead tissue from a wound to prevent infection and promote healing

Densitometry   the measurement of bone density

Disc (slipped disc)   the pad of cartilage between the vertebrae of the spine

Endorphins   chemicals produced in the body that reduce pain and increase the sense of well-being

Enteric-coated   a tablet coating that resists stomach acid, hence protecting the pill and delaying absorption until it enters the bowel

Enzyme   a protein that promotes change

Erosion   the process of eating away or wearing down

Extra-articular   (symptoms) occurring outside the joint, for example fever and malaise

Genetic markers   small differences in a person's genes that mark whether they are susceptible to a particular condition

Gluten   a protein found in wheat and other grains to which people can be intolerant

Gout   an inflammatory arthritis caused by uric acid crystals forming in the joint

Haemophilia   a sex-linked, inherited disorder (girls carry it; boys suffer it) that leads to potentially fatal bleeding because one of the clotting factors in the blood is absent

Histocompatibility genetic grouping factor contributing to what the immune system treats as 'self' or 'other'

Hypertrophy to grow abnormally large; the opposite of atrophy

Hypodermic under the skin; usually a needle

Immunoglobulins a large family of proteins, which includes all antibodies that attach themselves to antigens; part of the immune system

Immunomodulator a substance the modifies the action of the immune system

Immunosuppressant a drug that damps down the immune system

Inflammatory exudate a clear, gummy fluid which helps seal and heal wounds

Interleukin-1 a cytokine (chemical messenger) that promotes inflammation

Isometric exercise tightening or contracting muscles without other movement

Lyme disease a tick-borne form of arthritis very like RA

Lymph nodes (also glands) small bean-shaped sacks, part of the lymphatic system which runs throughout the body rather like the system of blood vessels; the nodes filter out bacteria and other foreign bodies and produce lymphocytes and antibodies

Lymphocyte a white blood cell; part of the immune system

Macrophage a 'scavenger' cell; eats up foreign or waste material

Metabolism the chemical process by which food is broken down and turned into energy or tissue, and waste products eliminated

Monoclonal antibodies man-made antibodies which target a specific harmful antigen

Neuro-linguistic programming/time-line therapy/emotional freedom techniques techniques for curing people of phobias or anxiety

Neutrophil white blood cell involved in inflammation

Nodules small, painless lumps that appear on bony prominences or tendons

Oedema pooling of fluid in the tissues; finger-pressure leaves a depression

Orthopaedic   surgery of the musculoskeletal system (literally, it means 'to straighten the child')

Osteoarthritis   degenerative joint damage caused by wear and tear

Osteoporosis   thinning of bone, loss of density that makes breakage more likely

Pannus   a thickening of synovial tissue that grows over cartilage and bone and produces enzymes that destroy them

Pericardium   the membrane sheath surrounding the heart which becomes inflamed in pericarditis, a serious complication of RA

Platelets   (or thrombocytes) small blood cells required for clotting

Pleurisy   inflammation of the pleura, the membrane sheath enclosing the lungs

Pneumonia   inflammation of the lungs

Prognosis   the most likely course of events; literally 'forward knowledge'

Proliferation   increase in numbers

Prostaglandins   substances that produce and modify inflammation, among other things

Prosthesis   an artificial body-part

Protein   the essential building-blocks of living systems, made up of chains of several molecules

Pseudo gout   an inflammatory arthritis cause by calcium crystals forming in the joint

Psoriatic arthritis   arthritis associated with the skin disorder psoriasis, characterized by raised, scaly, red patches

'Qualy'   short for Quality of Life measure; these attempt to quantify a patient's well-being and social functioning

Range-of-motion   exercises that extend an RA-affected joint's range of motion

Receptor antagonist   a drug that reduces inflammation by blocking the docking-site where pro-inflammatory cytokines deliver their messages

Reiter's disease   an arthritis accompanied by inflammation of the eye and urethra (the tube carrying urine away from the bladder)

Remission   when illness stops without being cured; not necessarily for ever

Retinopathy   damage to the retina (the image-forming part of the eye)

Rheumatism any painful disorder of joints or muscles not due to infection or injury

Rheumatoid factor antibody found in the blood of about 80 per cent of those with RA

Salicylate (acid) the active compound in aspirin

Sensate focus love-making behaviour that stops short of intercourse; words and caresses to rekindle desire; recommended by therapists for couples with problems

Sicca syndrome dry (sicca) mouth and/or eyes associated with RA

Sternum the breast-bone to which the front ribs and collar-bone are attached

Subcutaneous under the skin; a way of delivering an injection

Synovial joint (synovial membrane, synovia, synovium, synovial fluid) a multi-directional joint characteristically enclosed in a fibrous capsule filled with fluid and lined by a membrane, both affected in RA

Synovitis inflammation of the lining of a synovial joint

Systemic affecting the whole body not just one organ

Systemic lupus erythematosus an inflammatory arthritis accompanied by a skin rash that is sensitive to sunlight

Thrombocytopenia reduction in the number of platelets in the blood causing increased bleeding and slower clotting

Titre a measurement of quantity, for example traces in a blood sample

Tumour necrosis factor (TNF) a cytokine (chemical messenger) that promotes inflammation; a target for biologic medication

Uric acid excess uric acid in joints forms the crystals that cause gout

Vasculitis inflammation of blood vessels

Vasodilatation reflex expansion of blood vessels; opposite of vasoconstriction; the principal means of regulating blood pressure

Useful addresses

Research and support organizations in the UK

There are three major arthritis organizations in the UK; the first two are primarily patient-support organizations. The third, Arthritis Research Campaign (ARC), provides useful leaflets but also primarily sponsors research into the causes and treatment of arthritis. It currently has 66 projects running on RA at national centres of excellence all round the country (see Chapter 13, 'Hope for the future').

National Rheumatoid Arthritis Society
Briarwood House
11 College Avenue
Maidenhead
Berkshire SL6 6AR
Tel (helpline): 01628 670606
Email: enquiries@rheumatoid.org.uk
Website: www.rheumatoid.org.uk

Arthritis Care
18 Stephenson Way
London NW1 2HD
Tel: 020 7380 6500
Freephone helpline: 0808 800 4050 (weekdays, noon–4 p.m.)
Email: helplines@arthritiscare.org.uk
Website: www.arthritiscare.org.uk
Arthritis Care produces a newsletter called *Arthritis News*. Details from their website or phone 0845 600 6868. It also carries a list of support organizations in this country and worldwide.

The Arthritis Research Campaign (ARC)
Copeman House
St Mary's Court
St Mary's Gate
Chesterfield

Derbyshire S41 7TD
Tel: 0870 850 5000
Email: info@arc.org.uk
Website: www.arc.org.uk
ARC's website provides details of research centres and scientific information about arthritis. ARC also publishes leaflets and a magazine called *Arthritis Today*.

Less specific to RA but nevertheless useful UK contacts are:

The College of Health
St Margaret's House
21 Old Ford Road
London E2 9PL
Tel: 020 8983 1225
Website: www.collegeofhealth.org.uk
Represents the interests of NHS patients in the UK.

Dial UK (Disability Information and Advice Line)
St Catherine's
Tickhill Road
Doncaster DN4 8QN
Tel: 01302 310123
Email: enquiries@DIALuk.org.uk
Website: www.dialuk.org.uk

Disabled Living Foundation
380–384 Harrow Road
London W9 2HU
Tel: 020 7289 6111
Helpline: 0845 130 9177 (10 a.m.–1 p.m. Mon–Fri)
Website: www.dlf.org.uk

Organizations in Ireland, New Zealand, Canada and the USA

The Arthritis Foundation of Ireland
1 Clanwilliam Square
Grand Canal Quay

Dublin 2
Ireland
Tel: 01 661 8188
Fax: 01 661 8261
Email: info@arthritis-foundation.com
Website: www.arthritis-foundation.com

Arthritis New Zealand
Level 2
166 Featherston Street
Wellington
PO Box 10-020
New Zealand
Tel: 04 472 1427
Fax: 04 472 7066
Email: info@arthritis.org.nz
Website: www.arthritis.org.nz

The Arthritis Society (National Office)
393 University Avenue
Suite 1700
Toronto
Ontario M5G 1E6
Canada
Tel: 416–979–7228
Fax: 416–979–8366
Email: info@arthritis.ca
Website: www.arthritis.ca

Arthritis Foundation
1330 West Peachtree Street
Atlanta
Georgia 30309
USA
Tel: 001 404 872 7100
Freephone in the USA: (800) 283 7800
Website: www.arthritis.org
A massive website with information, news stories, the latest research, patient histories and details of local offices all over America.

The National Institute of Arthritis and Musculoskeletal and Skin Diseases (NIAMS)
1 AMS Circles
Bethesda
Maryland 20892-3675
USA
General website: www.niams.nih.gov/

Their consumer information website includes fact-sheets on a range of topics including exercise: www.pueblo.gsa.gov/cic_text/health/rheumatoid/rheumatoid.txt.

RA on the internet

Websites including those run *by* arthritis sufferers *for* arthritis sufferers; the first is where you can find Carol and Rick Eustice: www.arthritis.about.com

National Rheumatoid Arthritis Society
a charity website developed by an RA sufferer:
www.rheumatoid.org.uk

American Autoimmune Related Diseases Association
www.aarda.org

The Arthritis Trust
www.arthritistrust.org

Websites for specific problems
The British Pain Society, information on drugs, pain clinics and pain management programmes around the UK
www.britishpainsociety.org

Help with phobias can be found at:
www.anxietypanic.com
An interesting article on the subject at:
http://www.washingtonpost.com/wp-dyn/articles/A6594-2004Apr1-23.html

Details of how to use sensate focus may be found at: www.partnertherapy.com

Elsewhere in cyberspace

Useful information is offered by several major universities. They will show up in any general search for information on managing or research into RA.

Tips on internet searching

The internet is a source of such endless information that the only problem is sorting the wheat from the chaff. Some useful tips: the boxes at the side of the page are paid for, so may have an axe to grind. The suffix .org implies a charity or an organization whose primary focus is not commercial. The suffix .ac or .edu implies an academic or educational site, likely to be well informed but possibly narrow or esoteric in focus. Beware of jazzy, all-singing-all-dancing sites. They probably aren't serious.

If you aren't on-line, go to the public library and browse for free. There is information, support and the experience of other RA sufferers out there to share.

Further reading

*Author recommendation

*Carrie Britton, *Kids with Arthritis: a Guide for Families* (published in 2004 by the charity Choices for Families of Children with Arthritis and available from them at www.kidswitharthritis.org). This book won the 2004 ARC award.

*Gretchen Henkel *et al.*, foreword John H. Klippel, *The Arthritis Foundation's Guide to Good Living with Rheumatoid Arthritis*, Arthritis Foundation, 2000

Cheryl Koehn *et al.*, *Rheumatoid Arthritis: Plan to Win*, Oxford University Press, 2002

Robert Moots and Nigel Jones, *Rheumatoid Arthritis: Your Questions Answered*, Churchill Livingstone, 2004

Stephen A. Paget, Michael Lockshin and Suzanne Loebl, *The Hospital for Special Surgery Rheumatoid Arthritis Handbook: Everything You Need to Know*, Wiley, 2002 (also available as an e-book)

James N. Parker, *The Official Patient's Sourcebook on Rheumatoid Arthritis*, Icon Health Publications, 2002 (also available as an e-book)

Robert H. Phillips, *Coping with Rheumatoid Arthritis (Coping with Chronic Conditions: Guides to Living with Chronic Illnesses for You and Your Family)*, Avery Publishing, 1989

E. William St Clair *et al.*, *Rheumatoid Arthritis*, Lippincott, Williams and Wilkins, 2004 (this is a technical medical textbook aimed at clinicians, and priced accordingly!)

* Tammi L. Shlotzhauer and James L. McGuire, *Living with Rheumatoid Arthritis*, Johns Hopkins University Press, 2003

* Dava Sobel and Arthur C. Klein, *Arthritis: the Complete Guide to Relief Using Methods that Really Work*, Robinson Publishing, 1994 (second edition in 2005)

Index